CANCER MANAGEMENT

Edited by **Doaa Hashad**

Cancer Management
Edited by Doaa Hashad

Published by InTech
Janeza Trdine 9, 51000 Rijeka, Croatia

Publishing Process Manager Marija Radja

Technical Editor Teodora Smiljanic

Cover Designer InTech Design Team

Additional hard copies can be obtained from orders@intechopen.com

Cancer Management, Edited by Doaa Hashad
p. cm.
ISBN 978-953-51-0650-0

For EU product safety concerns:
IN TECH d.o.o., Prolaz Marije Krucifikse Kozulić 3, 51000 Rijeka, Croatia,
info@intechopen.com or visit our website at intechopen.com.

Meet the editor

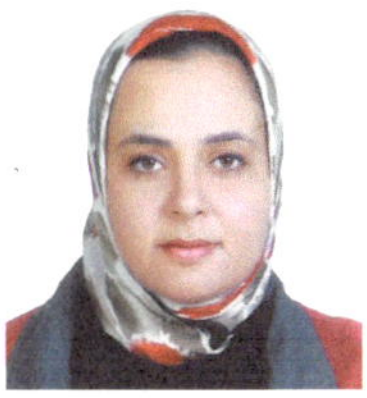

Dr. Doaa Hashad is an associate professor in the Clinical Pathology Department, Alexandria Faculty of Medicine, Alexandria, Egypt. She obtained her masters in clinical pathology in 2001 and her MD in clinical pathology from the University of Alexandria in 2007. Dr. Doaa Hashad has many publications to her credit in international, peer-reviewed journals concerning the use of variable molecular techniques in the management of different diseases.

Contents

Preface

Cancer remains a major clinical challenge as a cause of death due to its frequent poor prognosis and limited treatment options in many cases.

Cancer management book addresses various cancer management related topics including new approaches for early cancer detection and novel anti-cancer therapeutic strategies.

This book is a collection of studies and reviews written by experts from different parts of the world to present the most up-to-date knowledge on cancer management.

Doaa Hashad,MD
Lecturer of Clinical Pathology
Faculty of Medicine, Alexandria,
Egypt

1

Association of COX-2 Promoter Polymorphism with Gastroesophageal Reflux Disease (GERD) and Gastrointestinal Cancers from Iran: An Application for the Design of Early Detection of Cancer and Providing Prognostic Information to Patients in a Clinical Setting

Firouzeh Biramijamal
National Institute of Genetic Engineering and Biotechnology (NIGEB), Tehran, Iran

1. Introduction

Cyclooxygenase (COX) is a key enzyme responsible for developing several inflammatory diseases that may lead to cancer. The COX is an enzyme (EC 1.14.99.1) that it alters formation of prostanoids, including prostaglandins, prostacyclin and thromboxane. This enzyme converts arachidonic acid to prostaglandin H_2 (PGH_2) which it precursor of the prostanoids. The COX enzyme has two active sites, including heme site and cyclooxygenase site. The heme site has proxidase activity that alters the reduction of PGG_2 (hydroperoxy endoperoxide prostaglandin G_2) to PGH_2, and, cyclooxygenase site converts arachidonic acid into PGG_2. It is described three COX isoenzymes, including COX-1, COX-2 and COX-3 (splice variant of COX-1). COX-1 is a constitutive enzyme and, it is expressed in most mammalian cells. Conversely, COX-2 is not expressed in most normal mammalian tissues, so, it is an inducible enzyme and it is increased in activated macrophages and during inflammation. Inflammation has central role for tumor progression. Presence of inflammatory cells can lead DNA-damage-promoting agents. Now, it is clear the relationship between inflammation and cancer. Macrophage can be produced Transforming growth factor (TGF-α), consequential, permeability of the blood vessel and endothelium is increased in the presence of inflammation and in response to prostaglandins which is produced by COX-2 enzyme. Therefore, in this microenvironment with inflammatory cells, the extracellular matrix degradation can be occurred. Disruption of communication between the epithelium and stroma can promote cancer. Induction of Vascular endothelial growth factor (VEGF) and angiogenesis are observed after growing tumor cells, and presence of hypoxia. So, tumor cells can be received nutrients for more growth, figure 1.

COX-2 gene expression is enhanced in chronic inflammation. During prolonged inflammation, known as chronic inflammation, macrophages are produced TGF-α which it promote tumor growth, consequential, hypoxia is observed in microenvironment of tumor

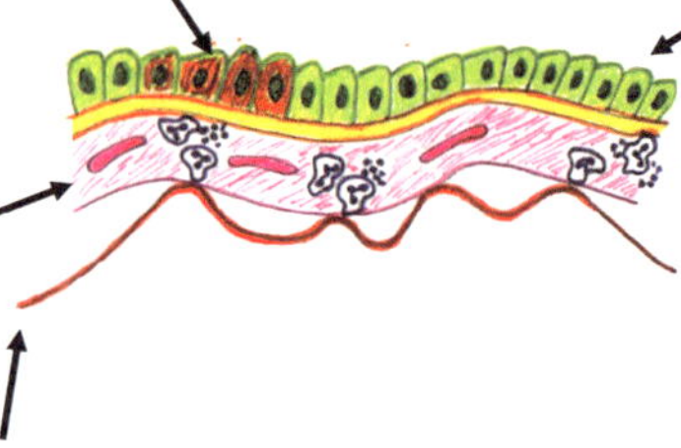

Fig. 1. Enhanced expression of COX-2 enzyme promotes tumor growth and cancer progression during prolonged (chronic) inflammation.

cells and inflammatory signals. Hypoxia is pushed the cells to produce Hypoxia-Inducible factor (HIF) which stimulates the release of VEGF. So, VEGF binds to VEGF receptors on endothelial cells, and leading angiogenesis. Also, matrix metalloproteinases (MMPs) upregulates in tumor cells microenvironment to degrade extracellular matrix proteins and tumor growth progression.

It is found that the COX-2 enzyme up-regulates in various carcinomas and it is described the role of COX-2 at an early stage in tumorigenesis. The COX-2 enzyme has been shown as an important mediator of proliferation through the increased formation of metabolites such as prostaglandin E_2. Also, it can be increased the formation of heptanone-etheno (Hε)-DNA adducts which are highly mutagenic in mammalian cell lines, and accelerate the somatic mutations which are detected in tumorigenesis. It is observed that somatic mutations could be arised about 80% of various cancers.

Enhanced expression of COX-2 has been reported in many types of cancer including breast, colon, lung, pancreas, prostate, esophageal during prolonged inflammation, chronic inflammation. So, COX-2 is involved in mechanisms of carcinogenesis. COX-2 expression and activity is induced by inflammatory signals and carcinogens. COX-2 overexpression is associated with cancer development. The COX-2 gene is located at 1q25.2-q25.3.

The promoter region of the COX-2 gene consists of various transcriptional regulatory elements including stimulatory protein 1 (Sp1) binding site. The COX-2 promoter variation alters putatively functional transcription factor-binding sites. A variant at position -765 G→C in promoter of COX-2 gene is involved in modification of COX-2 gene expression. Additionally, COX-2 -765G→C genetic variation is linked to change the level of gene expression and serum concentrations of C-reactive protein and prostaglandin E_2, and, inflammatory response is different among individuals with varient alleles, figure 2.

We describe in this investigation the role of COX-2 genetic variation at -765 of promoter region on the risk of gastrointestinal cancers, and also, gastroesophageal reflux (GERD) as a risk factor for developing Barrett's esophagus and then esophageal adenocarcinoma.

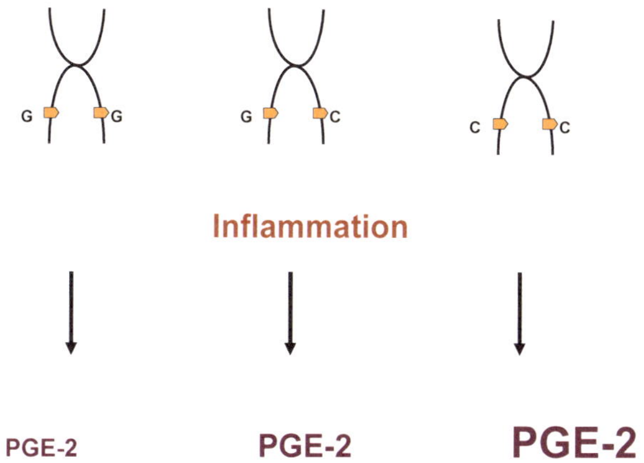

Fig. 2. Inflammatory response is different among individuals with varient alleles for COX-2 gene. The G→C substitution at -765 promoter of COX-2 gene can be changed gene expression and level of serun concentration of PGE_2.

Colorectal and esophageal cancers are frequent tumor types in gastrointestinal tract cancers. The COX-2 enzyme is known to be elevated in chronically inflamed tissues and gastrointestinal tumors. The COX-2 gene expression is dependent of interaction of nuclear proteins with the COX-2 promoter region. The promoter region of the COX-2 gene plays an important role in gene transcription. The single nucleotide polymorphisms in the COX-2 promoter can modified the binding of nuclear protein and consequentially, the level of gene expression and it can be changed susceptibility to cancer including gastrointestinal cancer.

It is described that reflux esophagitis can be changed to Barrett's esophagus (BE), and then, the risk of esophageal adenocarcinoma can be elevated 30- to 125- fold. The gastric acid reflux is the cause of esophageal damage in GERD. One of the most effective risk factors for inducing Barrett's esophagus (BE) is Gastroesophageal reflux disease. Gastroesophageal reflux disease (GERD) has been reported as a common disease worldwide. During reflux in the GERD, induction of the esophageal mucosal damage can be occurred due to inflammation. Also, chronic inflammation can be caused of progressing chronic esophagitis and premalignant Barrett's esophagus. The over expression of COX-2 gene is during chronic inflammation. It might be developed BE and adenocarcinoma (ADC) of the esophagus.

Barrett's esophagus epithelium is a premalignant condition prior to esophageal adenocarcinoma (ADC). The level of cyclooxygenase-2 enzyme is high in BE epithelium. It is shown that COX-2 gene expression is elevated 5-fold in Barrett's esophagus and 16-fold in esophageal adenocarcinoma compared to normal esophageal from healthy individuals. Additionally, it is seemed that COX-2 protein expression in the esophagus is independent of the degree of inflammation. Also, it is suggested that over expression of COX-2 can be used as a biomarker for detection of development of esophageal adenocarcinoma related to Barrett's metaplasia. The over expression of COX-2 is associated with esophageal carcinogenesis, and, the condition of tumor aggressive is dependent on the level of COX-2 protein expression.

It is reported that the individuals with -765C allele of the COX-2 gene are susceptible to esophageal cancer (both SCC and ADC lesions).

In addition, chronic inflammation can be caused of esophageal squamous cell carcinoma (ESCC) in Iran against western countries. In previous studies, it is reported that overexpression of COX-2 is approximately 70% among esophageal squamous cell carcinoma (ESCC) from Iranian patients and it is associated with p53 mutations. That investigation demonstrated the role of inflammation in carcinogenesis of ESCC in Iran as opposed to western countries. Comparing with esophageal cancer especially ESCC, the incidence of colorectal cancer (CRC) is relatively low in Iran.

In this chapter, it is described the association of COX-2 promoter polymorphism with gastroesophageal reflux disease (GERD) and gastrointestinal cancers from Iran. It might be an application for the design of early detection of cancer and providing prognostic information to patients in a clinical setting. In the next pages, it can be find some results for this aim.

2. Materials and methods

For this purpose, blood and archival cancerous human tissues from ESCC and CRC samples, also, esophageal tissue samples from GERD patients were collected. This study included 43 formalin-fixed, paraffin-embedded (FFPE) tissues from patients diagnosed with ESCC who had undergone curative surgical resection at Imam Khomeini hospital, 17 colorectal cancer tissues from patients diagnosed with adenocarcinoma who had undergone curative surgical resection at Tehran hospital. Then blood samples from eighty-two patients with at least one of three important symptoms of GERD (heart burn, acid regurgitation, or dysphagia) and erosive reflux esophagitis as diagnosed by endoscopy at the Endoscopy Ward of Fayazbakhsh Hospital (Tehran, Iran) and from 103 healthy indivituals were selected.

None of the GERD patients had taken proton pump inhibitors and Nonsteroidal anti-inflammatory drugs (NSAIDs) during last 4 weeks before beginning of the study. All cases underwent treatment with omeprazole as a proton pump inhibitors (PPIs) at 20 mg twice daily for 4 weeks. At the end of treatment, second endoscopy was performed for all patients and second biopsy was obtained from the previous site.

The tissue samples from cancer patients were examined by a pathologist according to the pathological features of the tumors. Informed consent was obtained from patients and healthy individuals followed by completion of a structured questionnaire. Also, this study was approved by the National Institute for Genetic Engineering and Biotechnology. Hospital records were used to verify age, permanent residence, and ethnicity of individuals.

Genomic DNA was obtained from FFPE tissues in cases and from whole blood of patients and healthy individuals by the QIAGEN Flexigen kit or QIAamp DNA minikit (Qiagen, Valencia, CA). The extracted DNA was then kept in a -20°C freezer until further use. The COX-2 -765G → C genotyping was performed by PCR, and a fragment of 228 bp was amplified from DNA isolated from FFPE tissues and blood using the primers COX F: 5'-CATTAACTATTTACAGGGTAACTGCTT-3' and COX R: 5'-TGCAGCACATACATACATAGCTTTT-3'. PCR was performed in a 25-µl volume containing 100 ng DNA template, 50 pmol each primer, 10 mM each dNTP, 2.5 µl Q solution buffer, and 2.5 µl coral buffer, 1 U/ µl Taq DNA polymerase (HotStarTaq Plus PCR kit from Qiagen). Initial denaturation for 10 min at 94°C was followed by 35 three-step cycles at 94°C for 30 s, at 56°C for 30 s, and at 72°C for 30 s. The PCR products were subsequently digested with 10 U SsiI (Fermentas, Lithuania) for 3 h at 37°C and separated on a 3% agarose gel. If the CC genotype does not cut the PCR product, then there is a 228-bp fragment. If there is a GC, there is a cut site, and theoretically it should yield a 228 bp + 168 and 60 bp fragment. The GG genotype should give only a 168-bp and 60-bp fragment, figures 3 & 4. To confirm the result of PCR-RFLP, selected PCR products were subjected to DNA sequence analysis, figure 5.

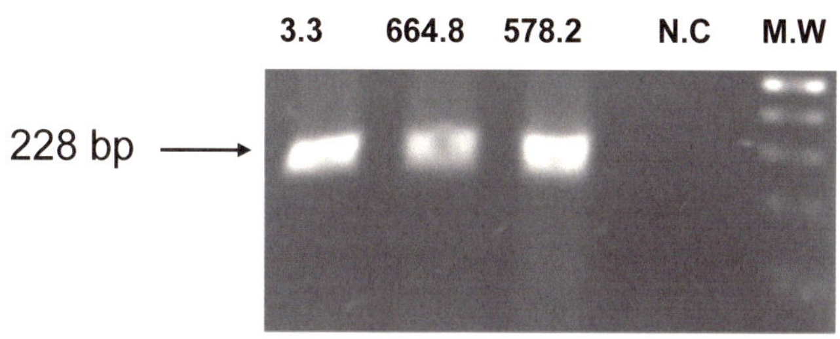

(a)

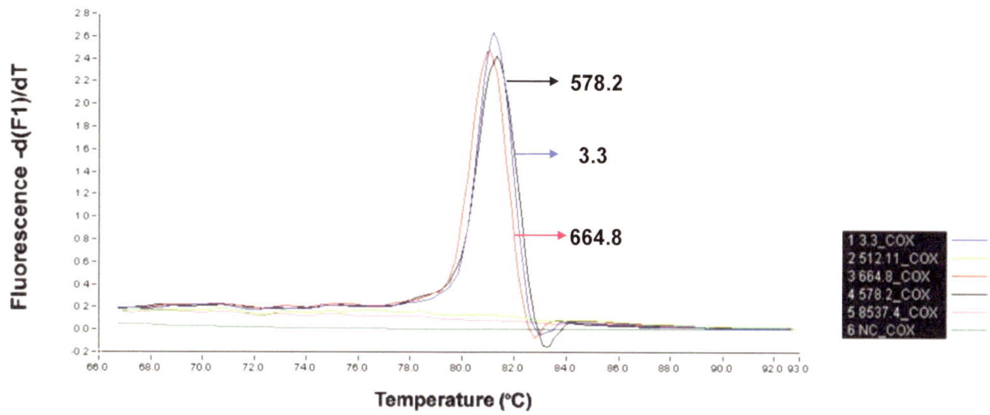

(b)

Fig. 3. A PCR assay to detect genetic polymorphism at the COX-2 promoter region. A 228 bp region of genomic DNA flanking -765 of promoter was amplified using primers which were described in the text. (A) The PCR products run on 2% agarose gel for cases numbers 3.3, 664.8, and 578.2 which were compared with negative control (NA), PCR reaction without using genomic DNA to control analysis and possibility of contamination, and a Molecular Weight marker (MW). (B) Detection of peak of PCR product with light cycler instrument to confirm exact amplification.

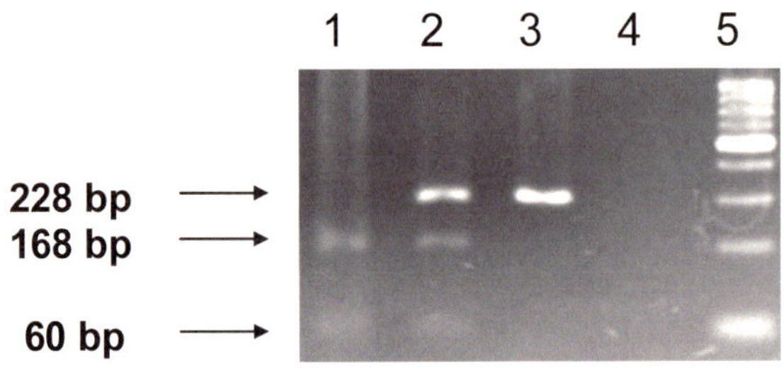

Fig. 4. Running digested PCR product with SsiI restriction enzyme on 3% agarose gel to detect of COX-2 polymorphism at -765 of the promoter region. Lane 1, sample with condition of homozygous genotype (G/G); Lane 2, sample with condition of heterozygous genotype (G/C); Lane 3, sample with condition of homozygous genotype (C/C); Lane 4, negative control (NA) to control the condition of digestion procedure using a reaction without restriction enzyme; Lane 5, Molecular Weight marker (MW).

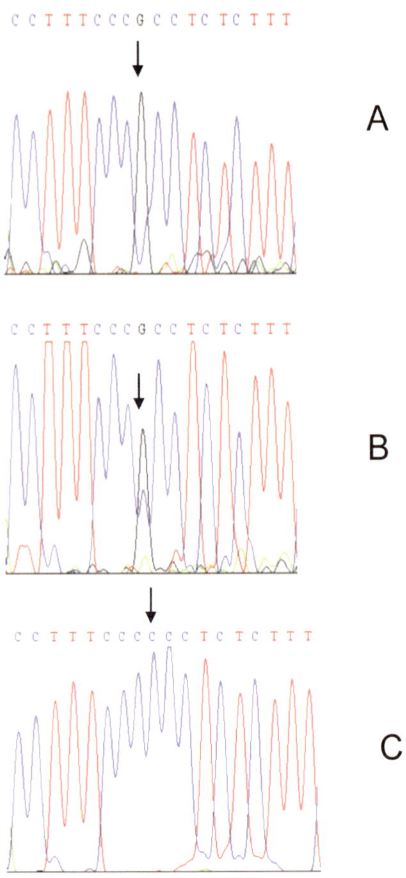

Fig. 5. Electropherogram of DNA sequencing (5′→3′) showing a single base substitution (G→C) polymorphism at nucleotide -765 of promoter region. (A) homozygous wild genotype (G/G). (B) heterozygous genotype (G/C). (C) homozygous genotype (C/C).

Of the 82 esophagitis tissue samples examined in this study for the COX-2 genetic polymorphism, frozen samples of 19 patients were available for evaluation of mRNA expression for COX-2 gene. The tissues were taken from GERD patients by endoscopic biopsy, and then, the samples immersed in RNA later (QIAGEN, Valencia, CA) for RNA preservation, where the tissue-containing tubes were kept in a -70°C freezer for later use. RNA extraction was performed by the QIAGEN RNeasy Kit, and the RNA samples were kept at -70°C.

For analysis of COX-2 gene expression we used real-time PCR method by Roche Lightcycler apparatus. Real-time PCR were carried out in a 25-µl. Reaction volume in Roche capillaries. The reaction mixture contains 0.5 µl TaKaRa Ex.taq and 12.5 µl TaKaRa one step Master mix, and 0.5 µl TaKaRa RT primers and 7.5 µl TaKaRa RNase free distilled water and forward and reverse COX-2 RT primers, each one 10 pmoL, and 2 µL tissue total RNA containing 250 ng total tissue mRNA. For internal control, we used β-actin for normalizing the expression values between all samples and obtaining comparative expression values relative to β-actin. Primers for the reactions were COX-2 forward: 5′-CCTTCCTCCTGTGCCTGATG -3′ and reverse: 5′-ACAATCTCATTTGAATCAGGAAGCT-3′, and for β actin: forward: 5′-GAGACCTTCAACACCCCAGCC-3′ and reverse: 5′-AGACGCAGGATGGCATGGG-3′. For each of the real-time amplifications, we prepared a standard curve by running real-time PCR with five 10-fold diluted cDNAs as template for COX-2 and β-actin, separately. Therefore, in each run for samples we had reactions for COX-2 and β-actin for every sample and one standard sample for COX-2, one standard sample for β-actin, and also a negative control for COX-2 and a negative control for β-actin. COX-2 to β-actin comparative values were obtained as final expression values for each of the tumor tissues and the normal tissues, both for cases and healthy controls. COX-2 real-time program consisted of three phases; a reverse transcription phase for 5-10 min at 42°C, then an amplification-quantification phase of 50 cycles of one denaturation step at 95°C for 5 s and one elongation step at 60°C for 35 s, and a final phase of melting by increasing the temperature from 65°C to 100°C in 15 s.

The *P* values of COX-2 genotype comparisons between cases and control groups were considered statistically significant and were below 0.05. This measurement was made by x^2 and Fisher's exact test. SPSS version 16 was used for all statistical analyses.

For comparison of COX-2 gene expression means, it is used the Student t-test, and ANOVA was applied for comparison of multiple groups in regard to their quantitative expression levels.

3. Results

Detection of COX-2 genotype for Cases (ESCC, CRC, and GERD/Control)

We investigated the role of COX-2 -765G→C polymorphism in a case–control study to find the distribution of allele frequencies. This polymorphism is known to modulate the transcriptional activity and expression of the gene. The study group of 142 patients included 43 ESCC, 17 colorectal cancers and 82 GERD genotyped for COX-2 polymorphism data. We assayed DNA from these samples for the frequency of allelic polymorphism at position -765G→C in the COX-2 gene. In healthy individuals, the distribution of genotypes fits the Hardy–Weinberg equilibrium. The frequency of the C allele was identical among the two groups of cancer patients (P=0.05), but the distribution of the CC genotype was different in the two groups (P = 0.001): 23.25% (10 of 43 patients) for ESCC and 5.8% (1 of 17 patients) for colorectal cancers. Our results showed that the frequency of the C allele (GC + CC genotypes of the COX-2 gene at position -765G→C among the cancer patients and GERD patients are high compared with controls. The variation of the allele frequency among cancer and GERD groups was significantly different from controls, P = 0.000, and P = 0.001, respectively.

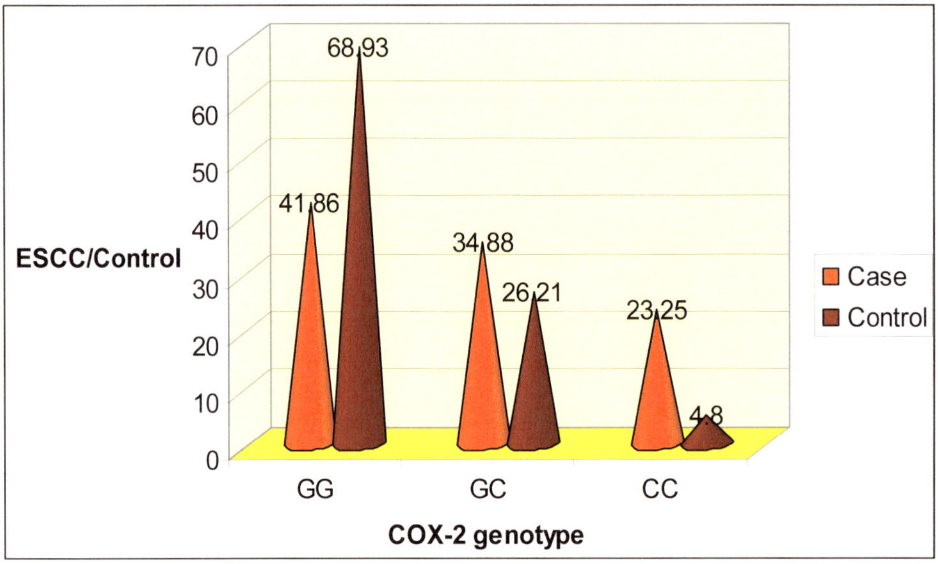

Fig. 6. Frequency of various genotypes of COX-2 gene among ESCC patients versus healthy individuals.

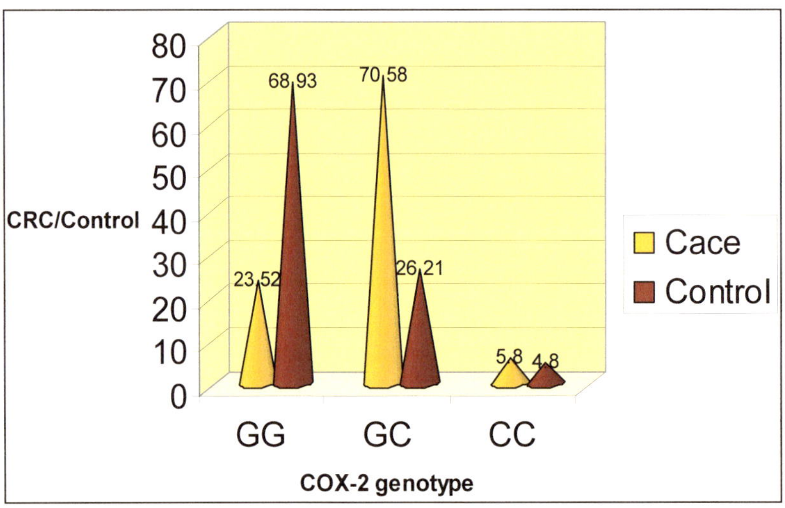

Fig. 7. Frequency of various genotypes of COX-2 gene among CRC patients versus healthy individuals.

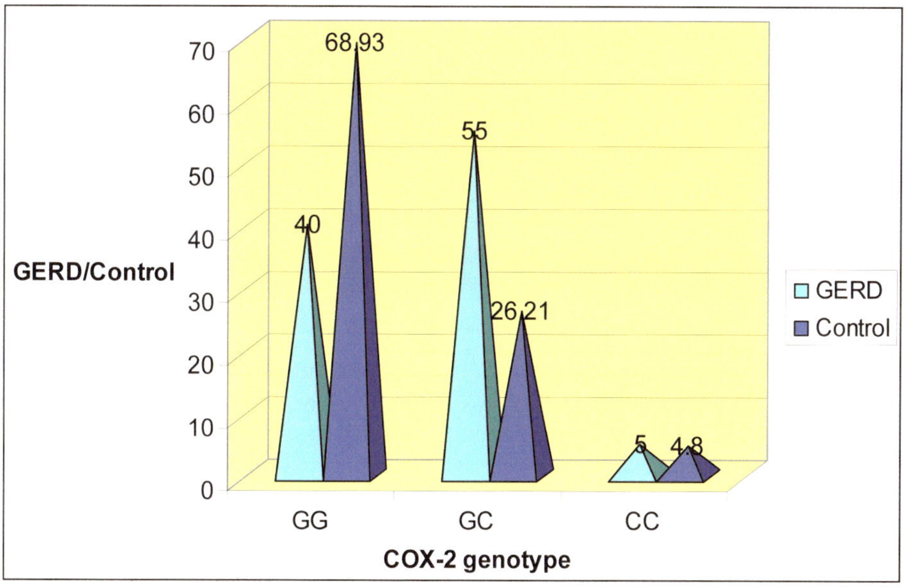

Fig. 8. Frequency of various genotypes of COX-2 gene among GERD patients versus healthy individuals.

COX-2 gene expression

Nineteen patients were enrolled in this study. We found that eight cases (42.1%) were -765GG (wild type), 10 (52.6%) were -765GC (heterozygous) and 1 (5.2%) was -765CC.

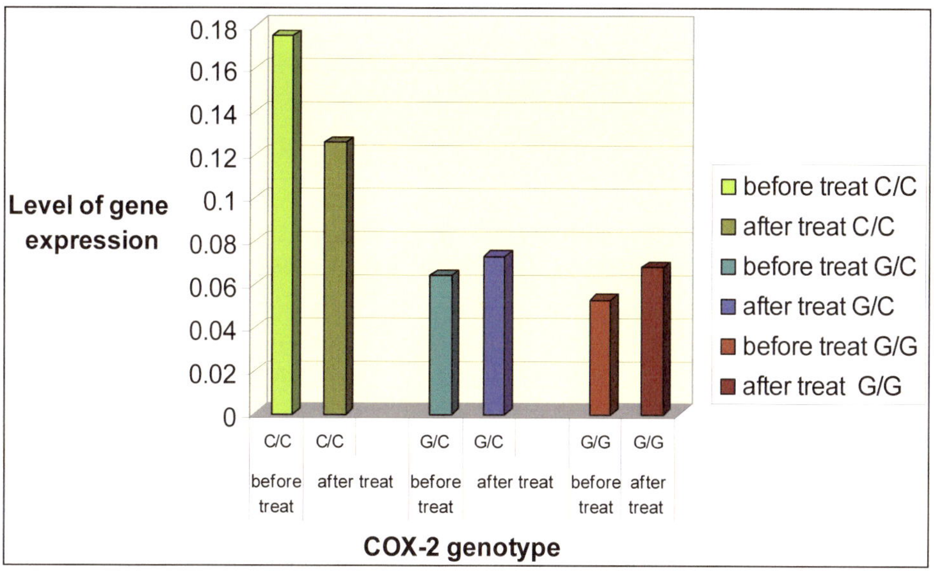

Fig. 9. Distribution of nucleotide variation at -765 promoter of COX-2 gene and its effect on level of COX-2 over expression. It is showed in this study that COX-2 overexpression is remained high among GERD patients after treatment with Omeprazole. It is assumed that C allele can be changed the activity of COX-2 enzyme against wild allele.

COX-2 mRNA expression was detectable by quantitative real-time RT-PCR in all of 38 tissue samples (were obtained from 19 patients in pre and post- treatment statuses). The over expression of COX-2 gene remained high after treatment with Omeprazole in the most of patients with GERD. The differences was identical among the two groups of investigated samples (P=0.07).

4. Discussion

The level of the COX-2 enzyme is elevated during inflammation, reflux esophagitis and in many types of cancers, including ESCC and colorectal cancer In addition, it is reported that COX-2 promoter polymorphisms can modulate the expression of the COX-2 gene.

Our results in the present study showed that the frequency of the C allele (GC + CC genotypes of the COX-2 gene at position -765G→C) among the patients is high compared with controls. This investigation could clarify the importance of the COX-2 variants in reflux esophagitis and gastrointestinal carcinogenesis in Iran. Our results show that C carriers are at higher risk for GERD, ESCC and colorectal cancers. In this study, it is found that the COX-2 over expression was remained after treatment period with Omeperazole in GERD patients with C allele at site of -765 promoter for COX-2 gene. Because, it is described that the level of cyclooxygenase-2 enzyme is high in Barrett's esophagus (BE) epithelium, and also, it is shown that COX-2 gene expression is elevated 5-fold in Barrett's esophagus, so, with regard of our results, it can be assumed that the risk of BE developing in the GERD patients with COX-2 over expression, after treatment with Omeperazole, might be occurred. This hypothesis must be investigated in further study according following up the patients.

It is shown that G allele at site of -765 promoter for COX-2 gene can reduced COX-2 gene expression. Additionally, it is observed that G allele can be changed serum prostaglandin E_2 (PGE_2) concentrations. Also, the COX-2 -765G→C polymorphism was demonstrated to influence the expression of COX-2 and change the risk of developing adenocarcinoma. Chronic inflammation can be developed epithelial hyperplasia, dyslasia, adenoma and adenocarcinoma in epithelium of colorectal.

It is described that COX-2 -765C allele is a protective factor against oral squamous cell carcinoma among Taiwan population. However, the COX-2 -765 variants has not effect on the risk of head and neck carcinogenesis among Netherland population. Our results showed that carriers with C alleles are at higher risk for Gastroesophageal reflux disease (GERD), Esophageal squamous cell carcinoma (ESCC) and colorectal cancers.

It is suggested that genetic variation at -765 of the COX-2 gene may change the over expression of COX-2 and therefore result in a higher synthesis of prostaglandins affecting the Barrett's esophagus and carcinogenesis process. In addition, it is described that -765C allele of the COX-2 gene affects carcinogenesis of ESCC in Iran.

Therefore, our findings can change the direction of future study, focusing on the use of therapeutic drugs to control and decrease the risk of gastrointestinal cancers among Iranian populations. Degree of COX-2 overexpression may be used as an inducible biomarker for detection of risk of malignant transformation in GERD patients.

5. Conclusion

It is suggested that identification of COX-2 gene expression and polymorphism at -765 of promoter can be used for design of early detection of esophageal cancer and providing prognostic information to GERD patients. Measurement of the degree of COX-2 over expression can be used as a biomarker for detection of susceptibility of malignant transformation among GERD patients.

Our study observed the association of the -765C allele carrier genotype with risk for ESCC, colorectal cancer and GERD in an Iranian population. Iran has a high incidence of ESCC in some parts (Golestan Province) and a young age distribution for colorectal cancer, and developing GERD symptoms. The results obtained from such studies can be of great importance from a therapeutic point of view, as both groups of cancer cells overexpress COX-2 and are more sensitive to COX-2 inhibitors. Further investigation of other cancer groups including ADC of the esophagus is required to compare with our results.

6. Acknowledgments

The author thanks Arash Hossein-Nezhad, Maryam Sadat Soltani, Guity Irvanloo, Kourosh Shamimi, Shaghayegh Basatvat, Nader Zendehdel, Nasrin Zendehdel, Masoud Doughaiemoghaddam, Hamid Reza Sarie, Akram Pourshams, Professor Reza Malekzadeh for their contributing in the projects which it redounded to writing this book chapter.

7. References

[1] Biramijamal F, Basatvat S, Hossein-Nezhad A, Soltani MS, Akbari Noghabi K, Irvanloo G, Shamimi K. Association of COX-2 promoter polymorphism with gastrointestinal tract cancer in Iran. Biochem Genet 2010 Dec;48(11-12):915-23. Epub 2010 Aug 31.

[2] Biramijamal F, Allameh A, Mirbod P, Groene HJ, Koomagi R, Hollstein M. Unusual profile and high prevalence of p53 mutations in esophageal squamous cell carcinomas from northern Iran. Cancer Res 2001; Apr 1;61(7):3119-23.

[3] Zendehdel N, Biramijamal F, Hossein-Nezhad A, Zendehdel N, Sarie H, Doughaiemoghaddam M, Pourshams A. Role of cytochrome P450 2C19 genetic polymorphisms in the therapeutic efficacy of omeprazole in Iranian patients with erosive reflux esophagitis. Arch Iran Med. 2010 Sep;13(5):406-12.

[4] Thiel A, Mrena J, Ristimäki A. Cyclooxygenase-2 and Gastric Cancer. Cancer Metastasis Rev. 2011 Dec; 30(3-4): 387-95

[5] Speed N. Blair IA. Cyclooxygenase- and lipoxygenase-mediated DNA damage. Cancer Metastasis Rev.2011 Dec; 30(3-4): 437-47

[6] Lisa M. Coussens, Zena Werb. Inflammation and cancer. Nature, 2002 ; 420(6917) : 860-867.

[7] http://www.wikipedia.org

[8] Brony S. Wiseman and zena Werb. Stomal effects on mammary gland development and breast cancer. Science 2002; 296: 1046-1049.

[9] Jason C. Fisher, Jeffrey W Gander, Mary Jo Haley, Sonia L Hernandez, Jianzhong Huang, Yan-Jung Chang, Tessa B Johung, Paolo Guarnieri, Kathleen O'Toole, Darrell J Yamashiro, Jessica J Kandel. Inhibition of cyclo-oxygenase 2 reduces tumor metastasis and inflammatory signaling blockade of vascular endothelial growth factor. Vascular Cell. 2011; 3:22 (doi:10.1186/2045-824X-3-22).

[10] Hilbert S. de Vries, Rene H. M. Te Morsche, Martijn G. H. Van Oijen, Iris D. Nagtegaal, Wilbert H. M. Peters, Dirk J. de Long. The functional -765GC polymorphism of the COX-2 gene may reduce the risk of developing Crohn's disease. PLoS ONE 2010; 5(11): e15011.

[11] Seung Won Jeong, Kyung Tae, Seung Hwan Lee, Kyung Rae Kim, Chul Won Park, Byung Lae Park, and Hyoung Doo Shin. COX-2 and IL-10 polymorphisms and association with squamous cell carcinoma of the head and neck in a Korean sample. J Korean Med Sci 2010; 25: 1024-1028.

[12] Simone P. Pinheiro, Margaret A. Gates, Immaculata DeVivo, Bernard A. Rosner, Shelley S. Tworoger, Linda Titus-Ernstoff, Susan E. Hankinson, Daniel W. Cramer. Interaction between use of non-steroidal anti-inflammatory drugs and selected genetic polymorphisms in ovarian cancer risk. Int J Mol Epidemol Genet 2010; 1(4): 320-331.

[13] Lin YC, Huang HI, Wang LH, Tsai CC, Lung O, Dai CY, Yu ML, Ho CK, Chen CH. Polymorphisms of COX-2 -765G>C and p53 codon 72 and risks of oral squamous cell carcinoma in a Taiwan population. Oral Oncol 2008; 44(8): 798-804.

[14] Peters WH, Lacko M, Te Morsche RH, Voogd AC, Oude Ophuis MB, Manni JJ. COX-2 polymorphisms and the risk for head and neck cancer in white patients. Head Neck 2009; 31(7): 938-43.

[15] Anastasia Papafili, Michael R. Hill, David J. Brull, Robin J. McAnulty, Richard P. Marshall, Steve E. Humphries and Geoffrey J. Laurent. Common promoter variant in cyclooxygenase-2 represses gene expression: evidence of role in acute-phase inflammatory response. Arterioscler Thromb Vasc Biol. 2002; 22: 1631-1636.

[16] Heather R. Ferguson, Christopher P. Wild, Lesley A. Anderson, Seamus J. Murphey, Brian T. Johnston, Liam J. Murray, R.G. Peter Watson, Jim McGuigan, John V. Reynols, and Laura J. Hardie. Cyclooxygenase-2 and inducible oxide synthase gene polymorphisms and risk of reflux esophagitis, Barrett's esophagus, and esophageal adenocarcinoma. Cancer Epidemiol Biomarkers Prev. 2008; 17: 727-731.

[17] M. Pawlik, R. Pajdo, S. Kwiecien, A. Ptak-Belowska, Z. Sliwowski, M. Mazurkiewicz-Janik, S.J. Konturek, W.W. Pawlik, T. Brzozowski. Nitric oxide (NO)-releasing aspirin exhibits a potent esophagoprotection in experimental model of acute reflux esophagitis. Role of nitric oxide and proinflammatory cytokines. Journal of Physiology and Pharmacology 2011; 62(1): 75-86.

[18] Kuramochi H. Vallboehmer D, Uchida K, Schneider S, Hamoui N, Shimizu D, Chandrasoma PT, DeMeester TR, Danenberg KD, Danenberg PV, Peters JH. Quantitative, tissue-specific analysis of cyclooxygenase gene expression in the pathogenesis of Barrett's adenocarcinoma. J Gastrointestinal Surg 2004; 8(8): 1007-16.

[19] Abdalla SI, Sanderson IR, Fitzgerald RC. Effect of inflammation on cyclooxygenase (COX)-2 expression in benign and malignant oesophageal cells. Carcinogenesis 2005; 26(9): 1627-33.

[20] J. Majka, K. Rembiasz, M. Migaczewski, A. Budzynski, A. Patak-Belowska, R. Pabianczyk, K. Urbanczyk, A. Zub-Porowiecka, M. Matlok, T. Brzozowski. Cyclooxygenase-2 (COX-2) is the key event in pathophysiology of barrettt's esophagus. Lesson from experimental animal model and human subjects. Journal of Physiology and Pharmavology 2010; 61 (4): 409-418.

[21] Yuan Liang, Jia-Li Liu, Yan Wu, Zhen-Yong Zhang and Rong Wu. Cyclooxygenase-2 polymorphisms and susceptibility to esophageal cancer: A meta-analysis. Tohoku J. Exp. Med. 2011; 223: 137-144.

[22] Jia-Li Liu, Yuan Liang, Zhen-Ning Wang, Xin Zhou, Li-Li Xing. Cyclooxygenase-2 polymorphisms and susceptibility to gastric carcinoma: A meta-analysis. World J Gastroenterol 2010; 16 (43): 5510-5517.

2

Prevention and Early Detection of Cancer – A Public Health View

Ljiljana Majnaric[1] and Aleksandar Vcev[2]
Dep. of General Medicine, Dep. of Biomedicine, School of Medicine, University J.J. Strossmayer Osijek,
Dep. Of Internal Medicine, School of Medicine, University J.J. Strossmayer Osijek,
Croatia

1. Introduction

Cancer is the second leading cause of death worldwide. According to the World Health Organisation (WHO), 12,5% of all deaths every year are caused by cancer (WHO, 2006). This is more than the total percentage of people who die from AIDS, tuberculosis and malaria, put together (International Union Against Cancer [UICC], 2007). Frightening fact is that deaths from cancer are projected to steadily rise. From about 7,5 million of cancer deaths, registered in 2005, this number will likely to reach 9 million, in 2015, and about 11,5 million, in 2030 (WHO, 2006). On the other hand, the knowledge about the causes of cancer and interventions to prevent and manage cancer are also growing up very fastly. At the current level of knowledge, it is estimated that up to one third of the cancer burden could be reduced if strictly implemented preventive strategies aimed at reducing the exposure to cancer risks, and another third of this burden could be cured if detected cancer early and treated adequately. The term "*cancer control*" was coined to unify public health actions aimed at implementing evidence-based strategies for cancer prevention, early detection and treatment, however adapted to different socioeconomic, cultural and resource settings (WHO, 2006). WHO and its cancer research agency, the International Agency for Research in Cancer (IARC), provide coordination and the leadership in these international actions (WHO, 2006).

2. Cancer as a common ageing disease; The risk factors paradigm

2.1 Cancer as a common ageing disease

Modern societies are characterised by a domination of chronic noncommunicable diseases in morbidity and mortality causes, including cardiovascular diseases, some cancers, chronic respiratory diseases, diabetes and dementia. This is partially a consequence of the decline in acute infectious diseases, due to improvements in life conditions, sanitation and medical care, and partially of the fast spread of modern lifestyles, due to urbanisation, globalisation and technology progress (Pearce, 1996, as cited in Majnarić-Trtica, 2009). Modern lifestyles include increased consumption of processed foods enriched in saturated fats and sugars, smoking cigarettes due to market orientation of tobacco industry, reduced leisure time, use of automobiles for transportation, and increased availability of electronic entertainment and communication media, all contributing to a sedentary lifestyle and weight gain (American Cancer Society [ACS], 2002).

To prevent diseases, it is necessary to identify and deal with their causes. In the case of chronic noncommunicable diseases, that means identification of health risks that underlie these diseases (Venkat et al, 2010; WHO, 2009). Most important, in this issue, is that a particular disease is caused by multiple risk factors and that, in turn, many risk factors are associated with more than one disease. So, by targeting certain risks, it is possible to reduce the burden of several diseases (WHO, 2009). This observation is in line with the results of the Human Genome Project showing that there is no specific disease susceptibility genotype, yet numerous genetic variants account for many age-related phenotypes (Collins & McKusick, 2001, as cited in Majnarić-Trtica, 2009; Yang et al., 2003, as cited in Majnarić-Trtica, 2009). That means that the symptoms and signs of common chronic diseases arise from the complex interactions, taking place over time, among multiple genetic variants and environmental risk factors, shared between clinically related diseases (Buchanan et al., 2006, as cited in Majnarić-Trtica, 2009; Yang et al., 2005, as cited in Majnarić-Trtica, 2008a). The main mechanism through which an organism responds to external environmental signals was found to be an epigenetic control of genome function in somatic cells (Jaenisch & Bird, 2003, as cited in Majnarić-Trtica, 2008a; Sandovici, 2008).

2.2 The risk factors paradigm

Importantly, when planning preventive activities, is to understand that each risk factor has its own causes. In fact, there is a complex chain of events enabling many entry points for intervention (WHO, 2009). In the proximity, there are more direct causes of the diseases. Factors located further in the back, act through intermediary mechanisms, to produce these proximal factors. Causally most distal factors have their background in social conditions and are hardly recognisable. However, if modified, these background causes are likely to have amplifying effects, by influencing multiple proximal effects (WHO, 2009). Keeping this in mind can help health workers and policy makers to realise that besides individually oriented preventive measures, population-based strategies are of the greatest importance if they want to reduce health risks in a community (American Cancer Society, 2002; WHO, 2009). That means that an individual choice, regarding health-related behaviors, occurs within a community context that can be either facilitating, or interfering with these behaviors. For example, in order to disseminate healthy diet and increased physical activity patterns, policy makers should implement multiple strategies at the community level, to ensure that all population groups have access to healthy food choices and opportunities for physical activity (American Cancer Society, 2002).

Another important fact is that there is no simple correlation between economic development and the shift in a major disease burden, from acute infections to chronic noncommunicable diseases. Namely, as economic development occurs, tobacco and alcohol use and obesity increase, followed by the burden of chronic diseases, in decades later. However, mortality and morbidity from chronic diseases do not start to decrease until very high level of social and economic development is reached (Derek et al., 2011). In other words, only at a high level of awareness about chronic diseases, governments and policy makers are likely to respond on negative trends in health behaviors, by using a range of policy instruments to revert these trends. It is not surprisingly then, that in the coming decades, the burden from chronic diseases is projected to rise, particularly fast in the developing world (Daar et al.,

2007). However, chronic diseases do not simple replace acute infections; rather, developing countries experience double disease burden, that have a huge negative impact on their economies (Derek et al., 2011; Daar et al., 2007).

By attributing known risk factors, including behavioural, physiological, occupational and environmental ones, to the total number of deaths, or the burden of diseases (measured in DALYs - years of life lost due to premature mortality and disability), it is possible to estimate of how much the burden of diseases is attributable to these selected risk factors (Venkat et al. 2010; WHO, 2009). Based on such analysis, it was realised that more than one third of the world`s deaths can be attributed to a small number of risk factors. The five top-ranked risks include high blood pressure, tobacco use, high blood glucose, physical inactivity and overweight/obesity. They affect countries of all income groups: high, middle and low (Figure 1) (WHO, 2009). When taking into account the fact that two leading world`s causes of death include cardiovascular diseases and cancers, this is likely to suggest that avoiding tobacco and obesity, and using regular physical activity, can provide the greatest potential to minimise cancer risk (American Cancer Society, 2002; WHO, 2009).

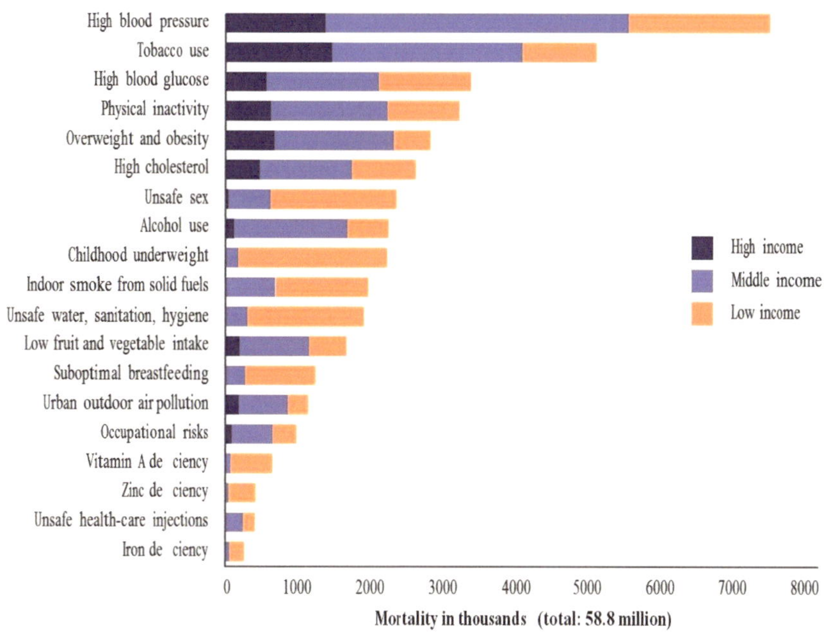

Fig. 1. Deaths attributed to leading risk factors, by country income level (2004)

3. Cancer with infectious origin

It is estimated that approximately 15% of all cancers can be attributed to viral infections. The oncogenic role of at least six viruses has strongly been established, including Epstein-Barr virus (EBV), Hepatitis B virus (HBV), Hepatitis C virus (HCV), several Human Papillomavirus (HPV) types, Human T-cell Lymphotropic Virus type I (HTLV-I) and Human Immunodeficiency Virus type I (HIV-I) (Boccardo & Villa, 2011). Cells infected by these viruses may turn towards oncogenesis after many years of infection latency, depending on the contextual, both the host-related, and the environmental factors - the fact that may complicate targeting potential preventive and therapeutic approaches (Butel, 1999; Weinberg, 1994). On the other hand, knowledge about the ways these infections are being spreaded on, is likely to provide directions for instituting adequate infection control practices. In relation to this, it is known that some of these infections are sexually transmitted and can be attributed to unsafe sex and non-use of contraception. Others are associated with using nonsterilised injection equipment, that is either related to unsafe health-care, or to opiates addiction (Boccardo & Villa, 2011; WHO, 2009).

The great opportunity for cancer prevention, at the global scale, lies in the development and distribution of antiviral vaccines (Schiller & Lowy, 2010). Commercially available HBV and HPV vaccines are already in use, and the major focus is now on their delivery, especially to low-income countries (Dempsey, 2010; El-Serag, 2011). The reasoning is based on the fact showing that HBV infection accounts for about 60% of the total liver cancer in developing countries, while for only about 23% in developed countries. For cervical cancer (HPV infection was proved as a course), the third most commonly diagnosed cancer and the fourth leading cause of cancer death in females worldwide, more than 85% of all cases and deaths occur in developing countries (Ferlay, 2010; WHO, 2009).

4. Environmental pollution and industrial carcinogenes

The discovery of smoking tobacco as a factor being strongly associated with lung cancer (more than 85% of lung cancers occur among smokers), has further emphasized the definition of other external factors that could probable cause cancer (that are termed "*carcinogenes*") (American Cancer Society, 2007, as cited in Majnarić-Trtica, 2009; Pearce, 1996, as cited in Majnarić-Trtica, 2009).

Accordingly, at least 150 chemicals and other agents, including ionizing radiation, occupational (workplace) and environmental airborne particles, some drugs, as well as foods and other consumer products, have been listed so far by IARC, as potential carcinogens (American Cancer Society, 2007, as cited in Majnarić-Trtica, 2009; WHO, 2009). It is estimated, for example, that occupational exposure to microscopic airborne particles accounts for 8% of lung cancer, that is the most frequent form of occupational cancer (compared to 12% of deaths due to chronic obstructive pulmonary disease) (WHO, 2009). The encouraging fact is, however, that the majority of occupational cancers can be prevented, through minimising exposure, substituting safer materials, and/or enclosing processes and ventilation. These all are measures within the domain of engineering manipulation, and policy and legislation changes (WHO, 2009).

Trends which deserve particular concern of the scientists, policy-makers and the public as a whole, are based on the growing number of evidence showing that long-term exposure to traffic-related air pollution is the risk factor which can contribute to overall and especially to specific respiratory and cardiovascular mortality in general population (Brunekreef et al., 2009). Even some consumer products, including food, cosmetics and household cleaners, owing to their overall use, are among the most significant sources of exposure to toxic and carcinogenic chemicals. Higher level of awareness is the first step to tackle more adequate legislation and adversiting options, as well as technology innovations (American Cancer Society, 2007, as cited in Majnarić-Trtica, 2009; WHO, 2009).

5. Global cancer statistics and calls for action

5.1 Global cancer statistics

Based on the GLOBOCAN estimates, about 12,7 million cancer cases and 7,6 million cancer deaths occured worldwide in 2008 and this trend continues to rise (Jemal et al., 2011). Proposed major reasons include: 1) the ageing, alongside with growth, of the world population, as cancer affects older adults at the highest rates, and 2) an increasing adoption of cancer-causing behaviors, due to the processes of modernisation and globalisation (Jemal et al., 2011; WHO, 2009). Of this total cancer burden, 56% of the cases and 64% of the deaths have occured in the economically developing world. Although overall cancer incidence rates in the developing countries are half those registred in the developed world, the cancer mortality is generally similar (Jemal et al., 2011). The main reason for this dysproportion is in cancer survival rates, which tend to be poor in developing countries, mostly because of a late stage at diagnosis and limited access to timely and standard treatment (American Cancer Society, 2007, as cited in Majnarić-Trtica, 2008b; Jemal et al., 2011; Ebling et al., 1993, as cited in Majnarić-Trtica et al., 2008b).

The most frequent cancer site diagnosed in females worldwide is breast cancer and it is also the leading cause of cancer death, comprising 23% of the total cancer cases and 14% of the cancer deaths. In general, the highest incidence rates are registered in the most developed regions, although 60% of the deaths occur in developing countries. Brest cancer is now the leading cause of cancer death among females in developing countries, a shift from cervical cancer which held this unfavorable position in the past decades. The second and the third most frequently diagnosed cancers in females are colorectal and lung cancers, the reverse order in cancer mortality (Table 1) (Jemal et al., 2011).

Estimated Age-standardized Incidence and Mortality Rates (per 100,000) by Sex, Cancer Site, and Level of Economic Development, 2008

	Females			
	Developed countries		Developing countries	
	Incidence	Mortality	Incidence	Mortality
Breast	66,40	15,30	27,30	10,80
Cervix uteri	9,00	3,20	17,80	9,80
Colon & rectum	24,20	9,70	9,40	5,40
Corpus uteri	12,90	2,40	5,90	1,70
Liver	2,70	2,50	7,60	7,20
Lung & bronchus	18,60	13,60	11,10	9,70
Melanoma of skin	8,60	1,10	0,60	0,30
Ovary	9,40	5,10	5,00	3,10
Pancreas	5,40	5,10	2,10	2,00
Stomach	7,30	4,70	10,00	8,10
Thyroid	9,10	0,40	3,40	0,70
All sites*	**225,50**	**87,30**	**138,00**	**85,40**

Table 1. Leading cancer incidence and mortality rates, females, for more and less developed areas, world (GLOBOCAN 2008)

In males, the most common cancer site and the leading cause of cancer death is lung cancer, comprising 17% of the cancer cases and 23% of the cancer death (Table 2). Colorectal and prostate cancers are at the second and the third positions in cancer incidence and follow the same order in cancer mortality, with the addition of stomach cancer sharing the third position with prostate cancer (Jemal et al., 2011).

Estimated Age-standardized Incidence and Mortality Rates (per 100,000) by Sex, Cancer Site, and Level of Economic Development, 2008				
	Males			
	Developed countries		Developing countries	
	Incidence	Mortality	Incidence	Mortality
Bladder	16,60	4,60	5,40	2,60
Colon & rectum	37,60	15,10	12,10	6,90
Esophagus	6,50	5,30	11,80	10,10
Liver	8,10	7,20	18,90	17,40
Lung & bronchus	47,40	39,40	27,80	24,60
Pancreas	8,20	7,90	2,70	2,50
Prostate	62,00	10,60	12,00	5,60
Stomach	16,70	10,40	21,10	16,00
All sites*	**300,10**	**143,90**	**160,30**	**119,30**

Table 2. Leading cancer incidence and mortality rates, males, for more and less developed areas, world (GLOBOCAN 2008)

5.2 Calls for action

Based on the global cancer statistics, awareness is growing that a dramatic stride in fighting against cancer can be done only if initiatives are planned at the global scale. The framework for this call for a global action is provided in the form of basic documents, such as World Cancer Declaration 2006 (IUCC, 2006). According to this document, the aim is to increase the number of countries that have the national cancer control programs, including cancer prevention, early detection, treatment, palliative care and support for cancer patients. Cancer surveillance systems, including cancer registries, should be developed if they do not exist, to support data collection on cancer statistics, risk factors burden, and effects of measures done. Lower income countries will be especially encouraged to gain abilities for dealing with their growing cancer burden. In order to transfer the proclaimed aims into practice, international committees have established cancer control strategies (WHO, 2005, as cited in Majnarić-Trtica, 2008b).

5.3 The state in EU

In the European Union (EU27), 2,5 million of people were diagnosed with cancer in 2008 (Ferlay, 2010). During the past decades, cooperation at the EU level showed that it is possible to add value, beyond the national level, to reduce cancer burden in Europe. The goal, set under the Commission`s "Europe Against Cancer" programs (1987-2000), was a 15% reduction in cancer mortality by 2000 (Moss, 2000, as cited in Majnarić-Trtica, 2008b). Until 2003, the Program was at the half of this proposed pathway, with registered reduction of 9% (Boyle et al., 2003). Until 2008, some of the Member States, like Finland and Luxemburg and Austria, have yet succeed in their efforts to reach this proclaimed goal (Cancer Society of Finland, 2010). The horizontal approach, aimed at tackling major health cancer-causing determinants, is being accomplished through documents such as "European Environment and Health Action Plan (2004)", set up in order to minimise work-related exposures to carcinogens and mutagens, and "the European Code Against Cancer" (2003), set up to promote healthy lifestyles (as cited in Commission of the European Communities, 2009).

In general, although significant advances have been made in cancer control, cancer is still a major public health concern in EU, accounting for 29% (3 out of 10) of deaths in men and 23% (2 out of 10) of deaths in women (the facts for 2008) (European Commission, 2011).

Nowadays, the situation is characterised with substantial inequalities in cancer control among Member States, that is illustrated with the fact that mortality from cervical cancer is nearly four times, and mortality from lung cancer, in men - over three times higher, in the worst performing Member States, than in the best ones (European Commission, 2011). In order to strengthen efforts to share information, capacity and expertise in cancer prevention and control, the European Commission has recently proposed the "European Partnership for Action Against Cancer", for the period 2009-2013 (Commission of the European Communities, 2009).

6. Preventive measures that can reduce the cancer burden

Based on the experience gained so far, it is considered that a substantial proportion of the cancer burden worldwide could be prevented if adequately implemented community-based programs for early cancer detection and treatment, tobacco control, cancer-related vaccination (for liver and cervical cancers), and health promotion campaigns (American Cancer Society, 2002; Commission of the European Communities, 2009; WHO, 2009) (Table 3).

• Implementation of principles of a healthy life-style, mainly by means of a healthy diet - low in saturated fats and carbohydrates and high in fruit and vegetable, regular physical activity, no smoking, and only moderate alcohol consumtion
• Changes in sexual behaviour (including the number of partners, partners selection, the type of sex involved, knowledge on infection status of partners, use of barrier contraceptives)
• Immunization against Hepatitis B Virus (HBV) and Human Papilloma Virus (HPV) infection
• Taking the control over occupational hazards
• Avoidance of cancer-causing substances in the global environment and in consumer products
• Avoidance of attentive exposure to sunlight

Table 3. Primary prevention measures (taken before any sign of a disease occures) known to deal with the reduction in total cancer incidence

7. Screening protocols

The curability of cancer can be relatively high if it is detected in the early, localised stage (American Cancer Society, 2007, as cited in Majnarić-Trtica, 2008b; Ebling et al., 1993, as cited in Majnarić-Trtica et al., 2008b). Results of randomised trials and experience of the countries where national programs for prevention and early detection of cancer have been implemented, showed that the implementation of such programs, especially when they are well prepared and monitored, is the most efficient and, in the long run, the least costly approach to fight cancer (Levin, B., et al., 2003, Nystrom, L., 2002, as cited in Majnarić-Trtica, 2008b). Based on these facts, respective agencies, such as the American Cancer Society, United States Preventive Services Task Force (USPSTF), WHO, and the European Union Advisory Committee on Cancer Prevention (EUACCP), set up recommendations for the early detection of cancer (American Cancer Society Guidelines for the Early Detection of Cancer, 2007, The Council of the European Union Recommendation of 2 December 2003 on cancer screening (2003/878/EC), 2003, WHO Program on Cancer Control, 2003, as cited in Majnarić-Trtica, 2008b).

In principle, these programs may be two-way oriented. One way is promotion of the early diagnosis by recognising the early clinical symptoms and signs of cancer, based on health education programs performed for both, primary health care physicians and the population (WHO/Cancer, 2007, Wender, R.C., 2007, as cited in Majnarić-Trtica, 2008b). The other way is screening of an apparently healthy population, before clinical signs of cancer are detectable, in order to find individuals with the early cancer or pre-cancer stages (Moss, S., 2000, as cited in Majnarić-Trtica, 2008b). In this sense, screening procedures are considered as measures of a secondary prevention. There are two main approaches for targeting population: 1) targeting high-risk people (with a lifetime risk of getting a certain type of cancer of at least 20 to 25%), who are most likely to benefit from the intervention, and 2) targeting risk in the entire population, regardless of each individual`s risk and potential benefit (WHO, 2009).

Fundamental for the screening is availability of effective (with the acceptable level of sensitivity and specificity), low-cost, simple for application, and safe tests. This is not possible for all cancer sites. Fortunately, screening tests proved so far as being feasible for wide implementation, correspond with some of the most frequent cancer sites. These tests include: high-quality mammography (for breast cancer), Pap cytology test (for cervical cancer) and testing for occult faecal bleeding (for colorectal cancer) (American Cancer Society Guidelines for the Early Detection of Cancer, 2007, as cited in Majnarić-Trtica, 2008b). The screening of prostate cancer by using prostate-specific antigen (PSA) testing has not yet been established routinely on a population base, although the increasing amount of evidence confirms that the early detection of this main form of cancer in men considerably reduces mortality, increases survival, and is likely to be cost-effective (American Cancer Society Guidelines for the Early Detection of Cancer, 2007; The Council of the EU, 2003, as cited in Majnarić-Trtica, 2008b; ESMO Guidelines Working Group, 2011).

Under the influence of the rapid technology progress and a large amount of randomised trials in which the validity of particular screening approaches have been assessed - screening methods and protocols are constantly being changed (Table 4) (American Cancer Society Guidelines for the Early Detection of Cancer, 2008). Efforts have also been made in looking for appropriate methods for the early detection of some other frequent and/or hazardous cancer sites, such as lung cancer, or pancreatic cancer (Harold, C.S., 2011; The Sol Goldman Pancreatic Cancer Research Center, 2011).

Screening Guidelines
For the Early Detection of Cancer in Asymptomatic People
Site Recommendation

Breast • Yearly mammograms are recommended starting at age 40. The age at which screening should be stopped should be individualized by considering the potential risks and benefits of screening in the context of overall health status and longevity.
• Clinical breast exam should be part of a periodic health exam about every 3 years for women in their 20s and 30s and every year for women 40 and older.
• Women should know how their breasts normally feel and report any breast change promptly to their health care providers. Breast self-exam is an option for women starting in their 20s.
• Screening MRI is recommended for women with an approximately 20%-25% or greater lifetime risk of breast cancer, including women with a strong family history of breast or ovarian cancer and women who were treated for Hodgkin disease.

Colon & Beginning at age 50, men and women should begin screening with 1 of the examination schedules below:
rectum • A fecal occult blood test (FOBT) or fecal immunochemical test (FIT) every year
• A flexible sigmoidoscopy (FSIG) every 5 years
• Annual FOBT or FIT and flexible sigmoidoscopy every 5 years*
• A double-contrast barium enema every 5 years
• A colonoscopy every 10 years
**Combined testing is preferred over either annual FOBT or FIT, or FSIG every 5 years, alone. People who are at moderate or high risk for colorectal cancer should talk with a doctor about a different testing schedule.*

Prostate The PSA test and the digital rectal examination should be offered annually, beginning at age 50, to men who have a life expectancy of at least 10 years. Men at high risk (African American men and men with a strong family history of 1 or more first-degree relatives diagnosed with prostate cancer at an early age) should begin testing at age 45. For
both men at average risk and high risk, information should be provided about what is known and what is uncertain about the benefits and limitations of early detection and treatment of prostate cancer so that they can make an informed decision about testing.

Uterus
Cervix: Screening should begin approximately 3 years after a woman begins having vaginal intercourse, but no later than 21 years of age. Screening should be done every year with regular Pap tests or every 2 years using liquidbased tests. At or after age 30, women who have had 3 normal test results in a row may get screened every 2 to 3 years. Alternatively, cervical cancer screening with HPV DNA testing and conventional or liquid-based cytology
could be performed every 3 years. However, doctors may suggest a woman get screened more often if she has certain risk factors, such as HIV infection or a weak immune system. Women aged 70 and older who have had 3 or more consecutive normal Pap tests in the last 10 years may choose to stop cervical cancer screening. Screening after total hysterectomy (with removal of the cervix) is not necessary unless the surgery was done as a treatment for cervical cancer.
Endometrium: The American Cancer Society recommends that at the time of menopause all women should be informed about the risks and symptoms of endometrial cancer and strongly encouraged to report any unexpected bleeding or spotting to their physicians. Annual screening for endometrial cancer with endometrial biopsy beginning at age 35 should be offered to women with or at risk for hereditary nonpolyposis colon cancer (HNPCC).

Cancer- For individuals undergoing periodic health examinations, a cancer-related checkup should include health **related** counseling and, depending on a person's age and gender, might include examinations for cancers of the thyroid, **checkup** oral cavity, skin, lymph nodes, testes, and ovaries, as well as for some nonmalignant diseases.

American Cancer Society guidelines for early cancer detection are assessed annually in order to identify whether there is new scientific evidence sufficient to warrant a reevaluation of current recommendations. If evidence is sufficiently compelling to consider a change or clarification in a current guideline or the development of a new guideline, a formal procedure is initiated. Guidelines are formally evaluated every 5 years regardless of whether new evidence suggests a change in the existing recommendations. There are 9 steps in this procedure, and these "guidelines for guideline development" were formally established to provide a specific methodology for science and expert judgment to form the underpinnings of specific statements and recommendations from the Society. These procedures constitute a deliberate process to ensure that all Society recommendations have the same methodological and evidence-based process at their core. This process also employs a system for rating strength and consistency of evidence that is similar to that employed by the Agency for Health Care Research and Quality (AHCRQ) and the US Preventive Services Task Force (USPSTF).

Table 4. American Cancer Society, Cancer Screening Guidelines (2008)

7.1 Screening of breast cancer

Breast is the most prevalent cancer site in women in both developed and developing countries, accounting for a quarter of women worldwide diagnosed with cancer (Ferlay, 2010). The incidence continues to rise, as the combined effect of mammographic screening, ageing of population, and some risk factors burden, including postmenopausal hormone replacement therapy, Western-style diet, obesity, and consuming alcohol and tobacco among women (Aebi, 2011; Warner, 2011). Although it is still the leading cause of cancer-related deaths in women, in most Western countries, the mortality trend has been decreasing in recent years, partly due to the screening programs implementation, and partly due to the improvements in treatment (Ferlay, 2010).

Risks Associated with Mammography	
Risk	**Comments**
False positive result leading to recall, with or without biopsy	Inversely related to age; for women 40 to 49 yr of age, cumulative risk at 10 years is approximately 49% in the United States
	Higher risk is also associated with
	Prior breast biopsies
	Family history of breast cancer
	Current estrogen use
	No prior mammogram or a longer screening interval
	Individual radiologist
	May cause short-term anxiety and psychological distress
	May have small but significant long-term negative effects on health behaviors and psychological well-being
False negative result leading to false reassurance	Little research has been conducted to determine the effect of this finding; in one survey, more than 99% of women stated that they would not delay evaluation of a new abnormal physical finding despite a recent negative mammogram
Overdiagnosis (and over- treatment)	Increases with age; a review of five random- ized trials showed an excess of breast cancers (both invasive and in situ) in all studies, accounting for 4 to 32% of cancers found by screening
	Screening programs and simulation models report rates from 1 to 10%, depending on age, outcomes included (invasive vs. in situ disease), country, and whether cases are incident or prevalent
Radiation-induced breast cancer	Estimated risk is 86 cancers and 11 deaths per 100,000 women screened annually from 40 to 55 years of age and biennially there- after; ratio of benefit to risk is 4.5:1 for lives saved and 9.5:1 for life-years saved
	Level of exposure to radiation with digital mammography is the same as or lower than that with film mammography

Table 5. Costs associated with mammography

It is estimated that over 90% of breast cancer in women can be cured if a disease is diagnosed in an early stage and adequately treated (American Cancer Society Guidelines for the Early Detection of Cancer, 2007, as cited in Majnarić-Trtica, 2008b). Several procedures are routinely used to diagnose breast cancer, including clinical (breast self-examination and bimanual palpation of the breasts and regional lymph nodes peformed by health care professionals), radiological (bilateral mammography and ultrasound) and pathological examination (based on the core needle biopsy). Some advanced imaging techniques, such as MRI (magnetic resonance imaging) and digital mammography, have recently been added, because of high diagnostic sensitivity of these methods (Warner, 2011). However, mammography is the only screening method to date proved as to can reduce mortality from breast cancer, and any other method can be used only as a supplement to mammography (Warner, 2011). For reading of mammograms, BI-RADS classification (stages 0-5) is used. Cases suspected on cancer (BI-RADS 4 or 5) are refered for follow up (Eberl, 2006).

Breast cancer incidence is strongly age-dependent, with only a quarter of cases occuring before age 50; less than 5% before age 35 (Ferlay, 2010). Based on these facts and on the results from randomised trials which consistently show a 14% to 32% reduction in mortality from breast cancer with annual or biennial mammography in women 50 to 69 years of age, screening mammography is universally recommended for women 50-69 years of age, with a 1-year, or 2-year screening interval (Nystrom, 2002, as cited in Majnarić-Trtica, 2008b; Warner, 2011). Some guidelines also include women aged 40-49, although data on the benefit to cost ratio have not yet been clarified (Table 4) (Mandelblatt, 2011; Warner, 2011).

Based on accumulated evidence, the decision to screen, more and more involves weighting benefits against costs (Table 5) (Warner, 2011). In the case of screening mammography, the most important benefits include reduction in the risk of death and the number of life-years gained. Costs include the financial costs and the by-products of the screening regimen itself (radiation risk, pain, inconvenience and anxiety), false positive and false negative results, as well as overdiagnosis (leading to overtreatment) (Duffy, 2010; Warner, 2011). The ratio of benefit to cost varies significantly with the patient`s age and depends on some other patient`s characteristics, such as breasts density (Warner, 2011). New, revised guidelines for breast cancer screening therefore tend to be more individually oriented.

7.2 Screening of cervical cancer

Cervical cancer is the third most common cause of female mortality worldwide, with the mortality rate 10 times higher in developing countries, and 80% of new cases occuring in these regions, compared to the developed countries (Ferlay, 2010; Haie-Meder, 2010). This disparity is in connection with low level of knowledge about unsafe sex and inaccessibility to screening and treatment programs, for women in developing countries (Ferlay, 2010; WHO, 2009). The main problem, in developed countries, is still insufficient coverage of women in the generative age with the screening test (Commission of the European Union, 2007; Haie-Meder, 2010).

Cervical cytology based on Pap smears remains the cornerstone of cervical cancer prevention programs, although this filed has rapidly been developing due to improved understanding of the natural history of the disease and technology innovations, such as liquid-based cytology, automated interpretation of Pap smears and testing for human papillomaviruses (HPVs) (American Cancer Society Guidelines, 2011; ESMO European guidelines for quality assurance, 2010). This, on the one hand, points up the neccessity for establishing the uniform indicators for monitoring program performance, to enable data comparison across the countries, and on the other hand - leads to fast exchanges of practice guidelines (Table 4) (ESMO European guidelines for quality assurance, 2010).

It is now well known that a persistent infection with sexually transmittable human papillomaviruses is responsible for virtually all cases of cervical cancer (Haie-Meder, 2010). Early age at first sexual intercourse and early pregnancies have been recognised as risk factors. The evidence linking HPV infection to cervical cancer has initiated the development of HPV DNA testing, to support more accurate risk stratification, beyond the capacity of conventional Papanicolaou smear testing (Figure 2) (American Cancer Society Guidelines, 2011; ESMO European guidelines for quality assurance, 2010). Also, primary prevention by prophylactic vaccination against the HPV types that are causally linked with most cervical cancers in Europe, HPV-16 and HPV-18, is now commercially available (Schiller & Lowy, 2010). The high efficacy of the vaccines is expected to dramatically decrease cervical cancer, by preventing up to 70% of newly diagnosed cases. However, prophylactic vaccination is performed in young girls and it will take a time until it provides the health gains. Therefore, cervical screening still remains the main preventive option (Figure 2). Nowadays, situation is that the high cost of the vaccine prevents its widespread implementation, which may further increase the gap in cervical cancer statistics between developed and developing countries (Haie-Meder, 2010).

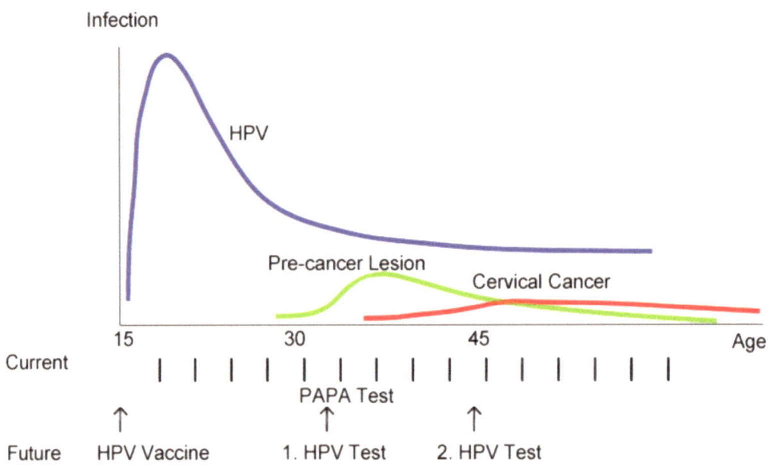

Fig. 2. Combined strategies to decrease cervical cancer

7.3 Screening of colorectal cancer

Cancers of the colon and rectum altogether are the third most common cancer type in the world and the most common newly diagnosed cancer in EU (Ferlay, 2010). In general, incidence is increasing along with industrialisation and urbanisation and is slightly higher in western and central, than in northern and southern and eastern Europe (Labianca, 2010).

Five-year survival rates, after the disease is detected, is much worse in the Eastern European countries, then in the developed countries (34%, compared to 54% and 65%, in the Western European countries and the USA, respectively) (Ferlay, 2010). As the result of the early detection programs implementation in many EU countries, in past decades, five-year survival rates show more favourable trends in all regions of Europe, compared to as it was before (Labianca, 2010).

Strong genetic influence can be attributed to only 5%-10% of colorectal cancers cases, due to either polyposis or non-polyposis syndromes, while the majority of cases occur sporadically (Balmana, 2010). The most important exogenous factors identified so far include: western-style diet and low physical activity, smoking tobacco and inflammatory bowel diseases, while the effect of chronic use of non-steroidal anti-inflammatory drugs for the prevention or regression of colorectal adenomas, has not yet been strongly confirmed (Labianca, 2010).

If take into account fact that a 10-35 years long-lasting period is needed for the transformation of benign adenomas to cancer, it seems reasonable to expect that the systematic implementation of the programs of active searching for subjects with localised cancer or pre-cancer lesions, could substantially reduce colorectal cancer mortality rate in population. It is estimated that under these conditions, colorectal cancer could reach a high cure rate of 80% and more (Winawer, 2003, as cited in Majnarić-Trtica, 2008b). This makes colorectal cancer an ideal candidate for screening. Since about 70% of patients are >65 y of age and the disease is rare under the age of 45 (2 per 100 000/y), target groups for screening usually include population aged 50-74y, with the minimum recommendations for the age range 60-69y (American Cancer Society Guidelines, 2011; Labianca, 2010). In order to complement community-based screening programs for breast and cervical cancers, established in many EU countries several decades ago, the EU Commision set up in 2003 recommendations for early detection of colorectal cancer, and the action plan "Europe against Colon Cancer", based on "the Brussels Declaration" (IUCC/Interantional Union against cancer, 2007, WHO/WHO Cancer Control Strategy, 2005, as cited in Majnarić-Trtica, 2008b).

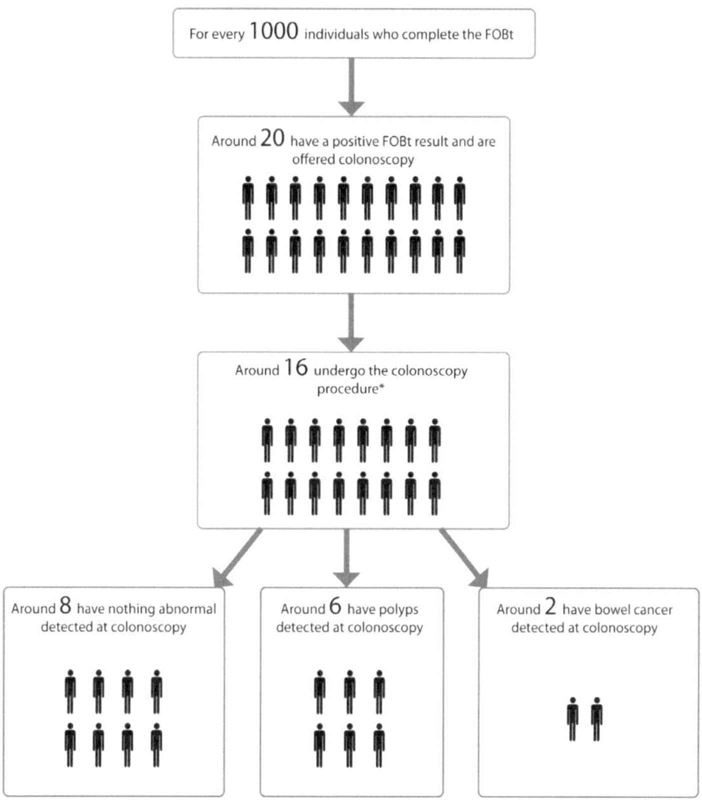

*Based on an uptake rate of 78%

Fig. 3. Predicted outcomes of screening on colorectal cancer (according to NHS.UK, 2011)

Up to date, two strategies have been available: faecal occult blood test (FOBT) and endoscopy (colonoscopy or proctosigmoidoscopy) (American Cancer Society Guidelines for the Early Detection of Cancer, 2007, BMJ Clin Evid Concise/Colorectal cancer screening, 2006, as cited in Majnarić-Trtica, 2008b; Labianca, 2010). Experiences on using the conventional screening method, the Faecal Occult Blood Test (FOBT), applied in asymptomatic population at average risk, showed that 3-5% subjects with positive results are to be expected (Winawer, 2003; Bond, 2006, as cited in Majnarić-Trtica, 2008b). The rationale for its use is based on the fact that, at an early stage, a colorectal tumour causes minor bleeding which can not be seen with the naked eye. The purpose of the screening is to check for this hidden blood in the stool sample. Recently introduced, the Faecal Immunochemical Test (FIT), has been shown as simpler for use and of a better specificity, however, because of higher price and the lack of efficiency analysis, it has not been yet widely implementated (American Cancer Society Guidelines, 2011). In most recommendations, the FOBT is used as a standard screening method, and a colonoscopy - for follow-up of test-positive cases. Based on widely obtained data, 10-15% of those subjects referred to colonoscopy are expected to be diagnosed as cancer and 30-40% as adenomas (Figure 3) (American Cancer Society Five-Year Relative Survival Rates, 2007, as cited in Majnarić-Trtica, 2008b; NHS.UK, 2011). Experiences until now showed that if screening strategies are implemented as organised programs based on the screening interval of 1-2 years, it is possible to reduce mortality rate for 18% -33% (Achkar, 2006, as cited in Majnarić-Trtica, 2008b).

7.4 Screening of prostate cancer

Prostate cancer is one of the three major cancer sites in men; commonly occures after 50 years of age, with incidence progressively increasing in later decades of life. Only males with positive family history of a disease (at least one blood relative: father, grandfather, or brother) are at a higher risk even in age before 50 (American Cancer Society Guidelines for the Early Detection of Prostate Cancer, 2011; ESMO Guidelines Working Group, 2011).

Screening protocol include digitorectal examination (DRE) and PSA (prostate-specific-antigen) measuring in serum, in patients aged ≥50 years, in those who refer symptoms of prostatism and urinary tract disorders, or in those who require screening. The decision on whether or not to have a prostate biopsy (performed by transrectal ultrasound, TRUS) should take into account PSA parameters, such as free (f) PSA, fPSA/PSA ratio, DRE findings, prostate size, patient age, comorbidities, patient values and history of previous biopsy (American Cancer Society Guidelines for the Early Detection of Prostate Cancer, 2011; ESMO Guidelines Working Group, 2011).

Although there are evidence indicating that population-based screening may reduce prostate cancer mortality by approximately 20%, patients should have an opportunity to make an informed decision on whether to be screened or not, since there are some uncertainties associated with prostate cancer screening (American Cancer Society Guidelines for the Early Detection of Prostate Cancer, 2011; ESMO Guidelines Working Group, 2011). Namely, screening increases prostate cancer incidence, including subclinical forms that will not develop during life, leading to unnecessary manipulation and overtreating. Long prospective studies, and cost-effectiveness and quality of life analyses, which are now under way, are expected to justify decisions on population screening on prostate cancer.

8. Programs of early cancer detection

In a general sense, screening program means systematic examination of the defined target population at average risk for developing some hazardous disease or undesirable medical event, or using scientifically justified tests that are appropriate to be applied as a public health measure (Table 6). Screening is organised periodically and at a long run, with the clearly defined aim to reduce the population burden of a disease and its unfavourable effects on the national health care system and economy. All activities in the program are fairly planned in an advance and performed according to the up to date standards of a medical care, with external finance assured. They include several subsequent steps, from promotional and educational activities, to screening, and a referal of subjects tested positive for further diagnostics and treatment. In concern to cancer, the early detection program is tending to become a part of more comprehensivelly shaped national strategies for cancer control, including also primary prevention and health promotion, as well as rehabilitation of cured patients, and palliative care for patients with infaust prognosis (WHO/Cancer, 2006). A programed approach has been proved as more efficient than the opposite one - an opportunistic approach - based mostly on patients demand, or performed in a diagnostic or clinical context. In the latter case, examinations may or may not be performed according to the public screening policy (Cancer screening in EU, 2007).

There is a wide consensus that a minimum degree of public responsibility, organisation and supervision, is required, for screening activities to be considered as within the context of a program, in opposite to a "non-program" screening. To qualify as a program, there should be a public screening policy documented in a law, or an official regulation, directive, or recommendation. As a minimum, the policy should define the screening test, the examination intervals, and the group of subjects eligible to be screened, including finance from public sources, or a co-payment. In a reality, substantially more organisational elements are needed to qualify screening activities as an "organised program". These elements provide for supervision and monitoring of most steps in the screening process, as well as comprehensive guidelines and rules to define standard operation procedures. In fact, differentiation of "organised" from "unorganised" programs should take into account the continuous gradient, ranging from poorly organised to highly organised programs. Further, a team, or the body, declared as being responsible for program`s implementation and coordination, can be organised at the regional or national level. Programs may be further differentiated as to whether they are population-based or non-population-based. Population-based programs generally require a high degree of organisation and that, in each round of screening, subjects from the taget population are individually identified and personally invited to screening. Finally, in the case of population-based screening, program implementation may be in various stages of development: planning phase, pilot phase, rollout ongoing, or rollout complete (i.e. fully established) (Figure 4) (Cancer screening in EU, 2007).

During last decades, evidence has been gained, in several countries in Europe, including Finland, Sweden, UK and Netherlands, which programs were performed to give possibilities for quality and effectiveness evaluation, on the benefits when implemented organised programs for early cancer detection (Cancer Society of Finland/Screening programme, 2011).

• the condition is an important health problem
• its natural history is well understood
• it is recognisable at an early stage
• treatment is better at an early stage
• a suitable test exists
• an acceptable test exists
• adequate facilities exist to cope with abnormalities detected
• screening is done at repeate intervals when the onset is insidious
• the chance of harm is less than the chance of benefit
• the cost is balanced against benefit

Table 6. Ten principles which should govern a national screening program (by Wilson and Jungner of the WHO, 1968)

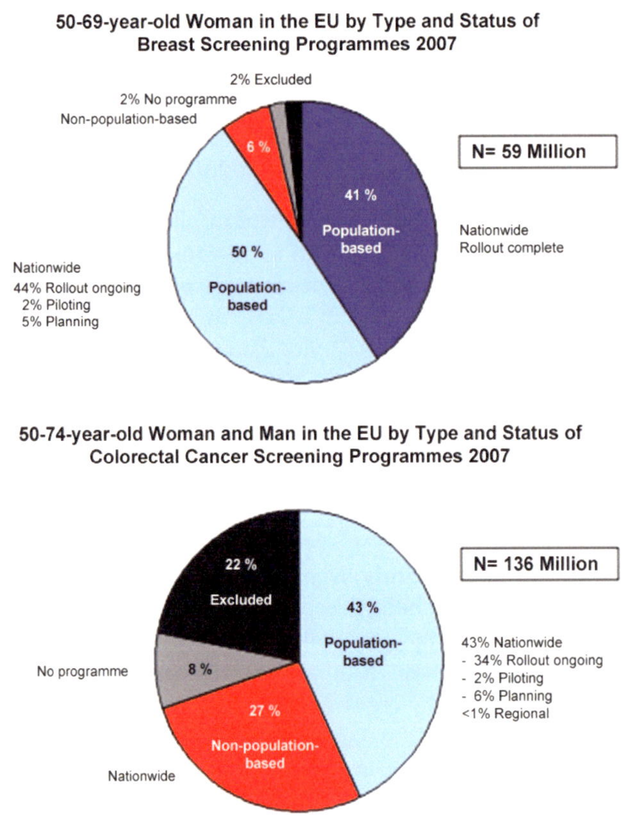

Fig. 4. Screening programs implemantation in the EU, breast and colorectal cancers, for usual target groups

Until 2007, 22 Member States (out of 27) have adopted policies aiming for implementation of population-based screening programs, 11 of them in which nationwide rollout of population-based programs is complete, 7 in which it is ongoing, and 4 in which it is being piloted or planned. Cervical cancer screening programs were running or being established in 25 of the Member States, but in comparison to the situation with breast cancer screening, program implementation varies more markedly and there is a substantial deviation from the recommendations of the Council of the EU. Compared to the prior two, colorectal cancer screening programs were running or being established in a smaller number of the Member States, program implementation was less advanced, and a smaller proportion of the population, specified in the Council Recommendations, was targeted (Figure 4) (Cancer screening in EU, 2010).

8.1 Programs of some European countries

8.1.1 Finland

In Finland, population-based cancer screening has a long tradition, as started in the far 1963 with cervical cancer screening (Cancer Society of Finland/Screening programme, 2011). Over the years, this program has come under the scrutiny, and now serves as a gold standard for evaluation of screening programs` quality and effectiveness. Two other main cancer screenings, for breast and colorectal cancer, are also being carried out in a highly organised manner. The first started in 1987, and the latter in 2004, after the EU Commission set up in 2003 its recommendations for strenghtening the efforts over early detection of colorectal cancer. The Mass Screening Registry provides evaluation of the impact of screening programs on cancer-related mortality and of the quality of the screening programs, and is a complementary to the Finnish Cancer Registry. The Finnish Cancer Registry is currently included in the European trial on prostate cancer screening.

Screening programs are centrally directed by the Cancer Society of Finland, but it does not exclude regional societies to work independently and to adjust programs to different local environments. These regional organisations provide a vast array of services, including counselling units, ambulatory cancer clinics, laboratories and hospices, as well as organisation of rehabilitation and recreational courses. Patient organisations and numerous volunteers, joined as members, provide the popular base to the Societies. The Cancer Society, together with the Cancer Foundation and the Foundation for Cancer Research, as private, non-profit investors, provide the sources of funds aimed at preventing cancer through research, health promotion and mass screenings. The Society also actively participates in creating health policy. In this way, the Cancer Society has become a vast forum for providing a support to comprehensive cancer control, by bringing together scientists, clinicians, decision-makers, financial experts, volunteers and patients, in the common mission of reducing the cancer burden in the population.

Specifically, Finnish smoking prevention and cessation campaigns, are worth meantioning details. Cigarette consumption in Finland was the highest in the world, in the period between two wars; consequently, the lung cancer incidence in men was one of the highest in the world. Due to combined effect of legislative measures, health promotion activities and strict monitoring, smoking decreased drastically over time, and nowadays is among the lowest in Europe.

By acting in this way, Finland has become one of the leading European countries in achieving an efficient cancer control, with the figures decline on cancer mortality and with the five-year survival rates among the best in Europe. Overall, in performing public health activities, Finland experienced a long process of transition, from the prevailing implicit policies, determined by commercial and fiscal interest, to explicit - health-oriented polices. In this context, earlier, the risk behaviour and a disease concern was considered as a medical and individual problem, while nowadays it is primarily considered as a public health, social and political issue.

8.1.2 UK

National cancer screening programs in UK include cervical, breast and colorectal cancers. For prostate cancer, there is an informed choice program - for healthy men who requires screening, and the risk management program - for men at higher risk for developing disease, due to symptoms of prostatism, or a positive family history on prostate cancer (NHS.UK, 2011). Cancer screening programs in UK are characterised with a high level of quality performance, and a large coverage of the target population, for cervical cancer already reaching the expected 80% (Arbyn, 2008, as cited in NHS.UK, 2011). Further, these programs are strictly evidence based, by means of the screening intervals, recommended age groups and methods used for screening. To avoid disparities for screening, community-driven approach is prefered, while Primary Care Trusts and regional directors of public healths are responsible for the quality assurance. The National Office for Cancer Screening provides the call/recall system and coordinate all other activities (NHS.UK, 2011).

The main shortage of this system is in using the lists of patients registered with general practitioners (GPs), allowing eligible individuals not covered by the health insurance, to drop out from the screening. The UK is an example of the cancer screening model which in a great part relies on the ordinary health care facilities and includes primary care teams to participate, by encouraging patients to screening and by keeping them informed on all the stages of the screening program. This model is termed as a "model service".

8.1.3 Hungary

Hungary, as a state in the process of transition, is typically faced with the growing burden of chronic noncommunicable diseases, especially concerning cancer (Kovacs, 2011, as cited in Hčjz/Health in Hungary). The life expectancy, of both men and women, is significantly below the average of most countries in EU, with cancer at the leading position in regard to "potential year of life lost" (PYLL). With the aim to reduce the overall mortality, and cancer mortality in particular, an organised cancer screening program, a part of the National Public Health Program, was launched in 2001. The official health care system is responsible for the program implementation, and finances are assured by the government. The program is coordinated and monitored by the Office of Chief Medical Officer.

Analysis made upon the program implementation, reveales some shortcomings, similar to ones found in other programs with small tradition. Some of these barriers to program`s implementation include the lack of necessary prerequisites for screening, insufficient finances, and a fairly high number of screenings performed outside the organised screening settings. The latter phenomenon may be due to the low degree of awareness for mass screenings, and to the fixation upon traditional examination protocols. Further, there is a poor cooperation among acters within the programs, the problem in record linkage, between various databases, and yet undeveloped laws on sensitive issues, such as data protection and patients rights (Kovacs, 2011, as cited in CJPH/Health in Hungary).

8.1.4 Croatian national program of prevention and early detection of cancer

Croatia is a transitional country characterised with health problems such as unhealthy behavior of the population and a growing burden of chronic diseases. The situation is even worse than it could be expected, because Croatia has recently experienced a war and fast political and social changes (Ebling B., 2007; Majnarić-Trtica, 2009).

In cancer statistics, in comparison with the majority of European countries, Croatia takes high unfavourable position (Draft National Program, 2007). Cancer is the second mortality cause and accounts for every fourth case of death. Both cancer incidence and mortality rates are on the increase, with a sharp increase in incidence rates observed after 1997, consequently to the post war period (Figure 5). The most common cancer sites are the lung, the colon and the breast, with the prostate cancer prevailing in elderly men aged 75 and more.

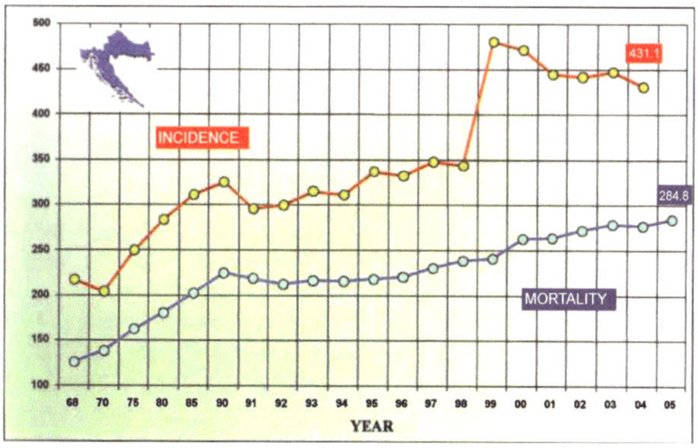

Fig. 5. Total cancer incidence and mortality rates, Croatia

In Croatia, primary prevention and early detection of cancer have not been systematically performed before, except for some separate actions, carried out by the non-governmental organisations or professional associations (Eljuga, 2006, as cited in Majnarić-Trtica, 2008b). The early detection of cervical cancer, by cervical cytology, has been performing for all sexually active women during their visits to gynecologists (Šamija, ed., 2000, as cited in Majnarić-Trtica, 2008b). Clinical examination on cancer and the FOBT have become a part of periodical medical checks, performed by family physicians for patients aged 50 and older.

Based on such situation and by taking into account unfavourable cancer statistics, the Croatian Oncology Society of the Croatian Medical Association initiated preparation of a Draft National Program for Prevention and Early Detection of Cancer (Draft National Program, 2007). The Program was published in early 2006. On behalf of the Ministry of Health and Social Welfare, the breast cancer screening program has started immediately that year. The National Program for Early Detection of Colorectal Cancer has started in late 2007. The Croatian Public Health Institute and its county departments coordinate and monitor program`s implementation, including activities such as the central call/recall system, data collection and evaluation. Family medicine teams are not actively included, only in keeping data on responsiveness of their invited patients to screening, and in follow up of those ones with positive tests.

General objectives, set up by the Program, are: to decrease prevalence of risk factors among the population by promotional and health educational activities, to reduce total cancer-related mortality rates by 15% within 5 years after the Program started, to increase the percentage of diagnosed pre-clinical and localised cancers compared to percentage of advanced stage disease and to increase the early detection coverage of the population. Specific objectives are oriented towards improvements in diagnostics and treatment and standardisation of protocols (Table 7).

CANCER SITE	RECOMMENDATIONS
Breast	• mammography for women aged 50-69, every two years • special protocol for women with family history of first-degree relatives with breast cancer, with determined non-tumour or tumour breast disease and other risks (earlier controls start, more frequent examinations)
Cervix	• Pap test for women aged 25-64, every three years
Colon Rectum	• Fecal Occult Bleeding Test (FOBT) or Fecal Immunochemical Test (FIT) for persons >50, every three years • Colonoscopy for persons with positive FOBT results to determine bleeding cause • Individuals at increased or high risk of colorectal cancer, including persons with history of colorectal adenoma or cancer, ulcerative colitis, Chron`s disease, family history of polyposis syndromes (FAP, Gardner, Turcot, Peutz-Jaghers syndrome, familial juvenile polyposis, non-polyposis colon cancer, first-degree relative with colorectal cancer should be included in early cancer detection program at younger age.
Prostate	• digitorectal examination and PSA test once a year for; - males at increased risk aged 40 years and older - males with prostatism symptoms aged 50 years and older; • males aged 50 years and older who request an examination
Health Awereness	• persons visiting family physicians should be distributed leaflets and brochures on prevention and early detection of cancer in the most frequent sites.

Table 7. Croatian National Program, Recommendations for screening

According to the Program for Early detection of breast cancer, women of the target population (50-69) are invited by surface mail to take preventive mammography every two years. Based on the planned coverage of 70%, it amounts about 280 000 women a year. BI-RADS classification and double-blind reading performed by two experienced radiologists are used as methods for checking up mammograms. Cases suspected on cancer (BI-RADS 4 and 5) are refered for follow up (Draft National Program, 2007; Ministry of health, 2006).

In the first screening cycle (until the end of 2006), about 720 000 women were invited, the number exceeded the planned number of 280 000 invitations a year, with more than 1500 newly diagnosed cases. (Experience from other European countries also showed increase in the cancer incidence during the first year of screening program implementation). Although achieved response rate of 58,5% was comparable to that in other European countries, the authorities are not completely satisfied with the results (Strnad, 2010). As the main barriers to program implementation, wrong addresses and insufficiently checked patients lists, were addressed. The rate of suspicious results was lower than expected, which indicates that women with BI-RADS 0 should also be taken into consideration for referal to diagnostics. Continuous education of radiologists in reading the mammograms and acquisition of new equipments for the diagnostic centres, are planned improvement measures. Educational activities, with the aim to increase the level of awareness for screening among the population, and further strenghtening the knowledge and companionships, as much among different sectors and participants included in the Project, as among local communities, will be essential (Samardžić, 2007; Strnad, 2010).

The screening protocol for colon cancer includes assimptomatic men and women aged 50-74 years, as according to the international recommendations, in two-year check-up by the FOBT, and the coverage rate of at least 60%. Test-positive individuals are referred to colonoscopy, to determine the cause of occult faecal bleeding. Individuals from the high risk groups are managed following the special protocols. Specialists colonoscopists and surgeons from clinical hospitals, and laboratory workers and coordinators from the counties` Public Health Institutes, are responsible for the Program implementation. Invitation letters are sent by mail to home addresses. In an envelope, there are three testing-cards, instructions for their use, questionnaire about risk factors and an educational brochure. Invited persons are asked to mail testing-cards back, after they used them, together with a filled questionnaire, the purpose of which is to obtain information on risk factors spreading in the population (Draft National Program, 2007; Ministry of health, 2007).

From the end of 2007 to the beginning of 2010, a total of 808 913 tests were distributed, of which only 19% were returned, 7,7% of these positive. Colonoscopy yielded 77,5% of pathologic findings, including 388 (5,99%) carcinomas; others were polyps (38,46%), hemorrhoids and diverticula (Strnad, 2010).

8.2 How to increase screening coverage?

One of the main problem, in mass screening programs, is how to increase the screening rates (*coverage*). This is two-sided problem. On the one side, there are problems of supply (program`s implementation performans), including necessary equipment, professionals, implement of evidence, establishment of the call-recall system, and strictly managed follow up (screening policy). On the other side, there is the problem of motivation of subjects from the target groups for screening (*patients` compliance with screening*). Two steps of the motivation process can be recognised: 1) a decision to enter the screening cycle (*up-take*) and a decision to stay in (*adherence*) (Flight, 2008; Smith, 2004). It is possible to affect patients` motivation (an internal mental process) by psychological transfer, including *patients` empowerment and education*, provided by physicians or other actors in the program (Masterson, 2006).

8.2.1 Promotional and educational activities

It has been recognised that the rate of up-take and adherence to screening may have a long-term effect on screening programs effectiveness (Smith, 2004) and that both processes, inherent in decisions for screening, are subjected to changes, by educational and motivational activities (O`Neill, 2008). This is why it is important that promotional and educational activities precede to and/or follow mass screening programs implementation.

Media campaigns and promotional activities can be organised at the national or the local community level, initiated by policy-makers, local community authorities, or public health services. These activities have multifaceted aim to inform the community on: 1) risk factors for the most frequent cancer sites, 2) early symptoms of a disease, 3) early detection methods, 4) the importance of acceptance of screening (Ebling, 2006, as cited in Majnarić-Trtica, 2008b). More focused educational activities, oriented towards specific population groups, such as high-risk groups, adolescents, or workers in industry, as connected with occupational risk factors exposure - can be initiated and organised by non-govermental organisations, local public health institutions, health professionals` associations, or cancer patients support groups (Eljuga, 2006, Ebling, 2006, as cited in Majnarić-Trtica, 2008b).

Individually-oriented educational activities, for patients` groups or individuals, can be mostly effective if performed by primary health care workers, especially family physicians. In the latter case, educational activities tend to be transformed into more subjective cognitive tools, close to what is known as "encouragment" and "empowerment" of patients for screening. In this way, some elements of a self-decision making process, connected with reasoning thinking, can be tackled to change (Fig. 6) (Ackerson, 2009). In this context, it is important to know that there are elements of a self-decision making process that are less prone to change. They come from intuitive thinking, complementary to more conserved psyhologic structures, such as the values and attitudes.

8.3 The role of family physicians in programs of early cancer detection

In terms of organization, two extreme early cancer detection program forms are possible, either that supplied by governmental and public health institutions, or that based on the central role of family physicians in program`s implementation. By working at the interface of the health care system and the population, family physicians are in the specific position that enables them an opportunity to promote a vast array of preventive activities, in a pro-active and a patient-oriented manner (Summerton, 2002). That means that the doctor recognises medical needs of the groups and individuals, encourages them to take preventive measures and manages the screening protocols, in contrast to the approach where the doctor generally responds to the patient`s requests. Moreover, the possibility of having an insight into specific characteristics of each patient, enables family physicians to select an appropriate way to present the preventive measures to a patient, and to create activities, in order to improve patient`s uptake and adherence to screening (Figure 6) (NHS.UK, 2011).

There is a general assumption that prevention and early detection of cancer is insufficiently implemented in practice of family physicians. In most countries, family physicians are only partially involved, mainly through opportunistic screening (subjects are referred by a physician for screening outside the program supplied by public services), or only under certain conditions, such as rural and distant areas (Moss, 200, as cited in Majnarić-Trtica, 2008; NHS.UK, 2011). Randomised studies in which screenings on cancer, managed by family physicians, were explored, are scared and not of a large-scale, to allow general conclusions to be drawn on (Jellema, 2010).

Decision Stages and Corresponding Physician Message	
Decision Stage	**Physician Message**
1. Never heard of CRC screening	1. Provide basic information about risk of CRC and benefits of screening
2. Heard of, but not considering CRC screening	2. Remind patient about risk and benefit of CRC screening. Discuss screening options.
3. Heard of and considering CRC screening	3. Assist patient to select a screening option. Help identify barriers and possible solutions.
4. Heard of and decided to do CRC screening	4. Discuss logistics. Ansver questions.
0. Decided against CRC screening	0. Probe for reasons and address them.

Fig. 6. Decision stages for colorectal cancer (CRC) screening

8.3.1 Experiences from Croatia in involving family physicians in programs of early cancer detection

The leaders of the Department of Family Medicine of the Osijek University School of Medicine and the Health Center Osijek, have recently introduced the project "*A Model of Early Cancer Detection Integrated in Practice of Family Physicians*", to test the idea that screening and early diagnosis of cancer are more efficient if integrated in practice of family physicians, compared to the National Program, centrally directed and supplied by the public services (Ebling/Project, 2007, as cited in Majnarić-Trtica, 2008b). The Project has started after two years of preparations and education of subjects from the target groups and family physicians, included in the Project, on screening and early detection methods. The computer program, specifically designed for keeping the records on data and for follow up of patients with positive screening tests, was installed into a total of twenty GP offices included in the Project. This program has allowed the continuous recruitment of new patients into the surveillance system automatically, by using personal data on sex and age only (Majnarić-Trtica, 2008b). Up to date, the Project has yielded its results in colorectal and breast cancer screening.

8.3.1.1 The Project of early detection of colorectal cancer

To avoid overalpping with the National Program, subjects were included in the Project for early detection of colorectal cancer to belong to either the 5-year lower age class (45-49) or the 5-year upper age class (75-79), than it is recommended according to the National Program (50-74). These defined target groups encompassed approximately 4 000 people, randomly selected from the large sample of a total of 27 000 subjects, recorded on the lists of family physicians included in the Project (Majnarić-Trtica, 2008b; Pribić, 2011).

The screening protocol can be described as follows. Family physicians call the patients from the defined target groups by phone, deliver them letters of invitation in envelops together with three testing cards, brochure for their use and a questionnaire on risk factors. A physician also provides instructions on how to correctly apply the testing cards and other issues the patients may be interested in. A physician reads the applied testing cards when patients return them back and keeps a record on the results. Patients with positive tests are referred for further diagnostics by colonoscopy. A physician also keeps a record on the results of follow up and treatments (Pribić, 2011).

From the beginning of April to the end of May 2009, a total number of 516 testing sets on occult faecal blood were delivered to patients from these two defined target groups. A high responding rate of 69,76% (360 cases) was recorded. This was an advantage in comparison with low responding rates of about 20%, obtained by the National Program. In the Project, there were in average 2,5% (13 cases) with positive tests, predominantely in the older age group, 3,5% (11 cases), compared to 1% (2 cases) recorded in the younger age group. These results showed that in the middle age population groups (45-49), a very low rate of positive tests, in systematically and non selectively performed screening on occult faecal bleeding, might be expected (1% positive tests). This further indicates that, for younger population groups, a selection of subjects at higher risk for the development of colon cancer should be made, prior entering the screening cycle.

8.3.1.2 The Project of early detection of breast cancer

The study group comprised the women from ten GP offices who have not yet been invited by the County Institute of Public Health to screening with mammography (Pribić, 2010). These women were invited during their visits for reasons other than mammography (opportunistic screening), or actively, by surface mail or phone. Women who did not respond at the first invitation, were included in the four-phased motivation program, carried out by a family physician and a home visiting nurse. If their decisions remaind unchanged after the period of three months of follow-up, they were classified as resisted the screening with mammography. Although a high level of responsiveness, of 80%, was achieved, a critical appraisal upon this study includes a suggestion for the post-hoc testing, to decide on whether a long-lasting and highly suggestive motivation activities are applicable as a routine advising procedure. In addition, results obtained here indicate, similar as in the case with the Project of early detection of colorectal cancer, that there is a need for more thoroughly prepared selection procedure, before someone starts motivating women to screening.

8.3.2 Concluding remarks

A central role of family physicians, in implementation of preventive programs, has been recognised as an advantage, in terms of achieving better screening coverage and decreasing the costs, as compared to the strictly centrally controlled programs. However, as with the respect to the above results - even those who advocate for this approach, must point out that some kind of technical and professional support to family physicians should be assured, to allow the program to maintain and to achieve high quality norms (Wender, 2007).

9. Current trends

9.1 Personalised screening

There is no doubt that the early detection of cancer is effective, but no clear attitudes on which strategy is more efficient than another, in a real situation within the framework of the current health care system organisation. Awareness has been increasing that variables such as "*a benefit-to-risk*" and "a *benefit-to-cost*" ratio, or „a *quality of life measures*", should be taken into consideration when planning screening strategies (WHO, 2009; Aebi, 2011). New, more specific screening tests, such as a digital mammography, or immunochemical tests for testing on occult faecal bleeding, are now available and increase our chance to detect cancer early. However, higher prices of these tests, compared to conventional ones, require more specifically elaborated screening strategies, including a precise definition of who should be included in screening, by using which tests, and under which conditions (Jellema, 2010; Schousboe, JT, 2011; Warner, 2011). Evidence also suggests that variables such as the patient`s context, including co-morbid health disorders, and patient`s values, regarding specific benefits and harms from screening, are to be taken into account (Warner, 2011).

9.2 Cancer risk prediction models

The average risk of getting a cancer (for a 5-years, or a 10-years time period, or expressed as a lifetime risk) are estimated on the basis of the incidence data for the population. Many factors that can change these estimates to the higher or to the lower, for some of the most common cancers sites, have been identified (known as cancer risk factors) (US National Cancer Institute, 2010, 2011). Knowledge on this issue allows personalisation of risk assessments, based on the estimates such as the score charts, or mathematical risk prediction models, which can help physicians and policymakers to identify individuals who might benefit, more than some others, from the screening.

Multivariable risk prediction models for some usual cancer sites have been established so far, based on using easily available epidemiologic and clinical data and identified risk factors. It has been realised, however, that the model`s precision can further be improved, if some biochemical or molecular biomarkers are added into the model or, more recently - information on a personal genome analysis (Barlow, 2006; Rosenbaum, 2010; Spitz, 2007, 2008; Wang, 2007). Risk prediction models are expected to support a decision-making, beyond the traditional screening protocols, by more accurately identifying subjects of the target groups.

9.3 Genetic risk estimates

Two Mendelian genetic tests, appropriate to add value to the cancer risk assessment, have been established so far, including BRCA1 and BRCA2, highly penetrant breast and ovarian cancer predisposition genes, and a set of the mismatch repair (MMR) genes, carriers of which have a high risk of the most common hereditary colorectal cancer and/or endometrial cancer, and a lower risk of urinary tract, small intestine, ovary, gastric, pancreas, biliary tract and brain cancers (Balmana, 2010; 2011).

The costs of the genetic tests were the main problem in the past, making the barriers for implementing these tests in routine practice. Nowadays, when the costs of these tests rapidly fall down, the dominant problem is a lack of the clinical assessments of genetic risk estimates. For example, higher prevalence of BRCA 1/2 genes can be found in association with a family history of breast or ovarian cancer and a young age at onset (Balmana, 2011). Is there an added value of systematic testing on these genes, in women with a positive family history of breast cancer, beyond the standard screening with mammography, if familial susceptibility to breast cancer accounts for less than 25% of all breast cancer cases? This further arises some additional questions. Namely, carriers should advise close family members to obtain genetic counseling and/or testing (American Cancer Society/A manual Cancer and Genetics, 1997/98; Balmana, 2011). This is associated with some ethical and moral issues addressing both, potential carriers and physicians who provide counseling for them. The major concern addressing potential carriers includes living under the pressure of having an increased susceptibility for cancer. Concerns addressing physicians include low level of knowledge on variation in penetrance and expression of cancer-prone genes, and a lack of evidence of how a genetic counseling might have an impact on issues from the ethical domains (American Cancer Society/A manual Cancer and Genetics, 1997/98).

9.4 The personalised approach in early cancer detection - the role of genomics and proteomics

The rapid progress in biotechnology has been expected to provide huge benefits in prevention and early detection of chronic noncommunicable diseases, notably cancer, by implementing genomics, proteomics and other -omics techniques in practice. The main principle, these techniques relies on, is a possibility of identifying subjects at an early clinical or subclinical phase, during the course of developing a chronic disease, by obtaining the whole-genome sequencing (genomics), or by characterising the protein and peptide profiles of various biological fluids or tissues (proteomics) (Yang, 2003, Khoury, 2007, as cited in Majnarić-Trtica, 2009).

These techniques have attracted the attention of both, the scientists and the public as a whole, in recent times, for their potential to stimulate the adoption of the personalised approach in medical practice, with expectancies for the improvements, equally in prevention, prognosis, diagnosis and treatment. For the reason that these techniques were developing far more rapidly than their clinical utility could be evaluated, there is no clear understanding yet, of what would be reasonable expectations of implementing these techniques in the real-life settings, and which obstacles need to be overcome. Although some early results of their clinical applications seem promising, such as the use of serum proteomics in screening for ovarian cancer, providing sensitivity of 100% and specificity of 95% - to date, there are no visible results yet, capable to bring substantial changes into the standard routine (Evans, 2010; Ioannidis, 2011).

10. Challenges for the future

10.1 Integrated knowledge translation

In spite of the huge advances in understanding the natural course of development of some common cancers, as well as in methods for their prevention and early detection, there are still difficulties in translating this knowledge into practice. The problem is especially emphasized in developing countries. Some of the main reasons include: separation between public health and clinical medicine, poor coordination between the health care and science - on the one hand, and the health care and politics and social welfare - on the other, and the rapid progress in health care technology and biotechnology, leading to a rapid rise in health care costs and the disparity in access. In addition, there is a need for better integration of the new, individually-oriented approaches into the established early detection programs (Evans, 2010; Hudson, 2011; Majnarić-Trtica, 2009; Pigeot, 2010).

There are initiatives to bridge these gaps, by favouring a collective approach to problems and questions concerning health. It is believed that this might be achieved through a leadership shift (from a traditionally top-down to a coalition leadership between practitionars and researchers/scientists), and the process of integration of the knowledge bases, among multiple health care and other social sectors. Namely, an awareness is growing up that the issues of public health are intimately embedded in the socioenvironmental context and should be managed within this context. For this reason, researches, public health professionals and policy decision-makers, should collaborate in searching for "better", "faster" and "cheaper" interventions, aimed at improving the health in the community. The development of the common information and communication technology infrastructure are expected to facilitate these common initiatives (Lapaige, 2010; majnarić-Trtica, 2009; Patridge, 2011).

10.2 The chronic care model

Improvements in the early detection, diagnosis and treatment of cancer enable people with cancer living longer and managing their cancers as a chronic illnesses. This consideres a long-term surveillance, including prevention, early detection, diagnosis, treatment, care after the treatment, and survivorship. Demands are put on patients and their families, in managing care on their own, and on family physicians, in providing them education and support, as well as a follow up (McCorkie, 2011).

11. Conclusions

Experiences gathered up-to-date show that the programs for early cancer detection are best performed if well organised and coordinated, independently on whether they are conducted by governmental and public health institutiones, or predominantly supplied by family medicine teams. In highly income countries, with long tradition in organising early cancer detection programs, expected curing and survival rates have been achieved. These favourable results can not be attributed only to a large number of professionals employed, good technical facilities and government officials coordinating the programs, but, even partially, to the comprehensively performed and sustainable driven strategies aimed at cutting the common risks factors burden for the most important chronic diseases, including cardiovascular diseases, diabetes and cancer. In this sense, the best way to invest in populations` health, would be by ensuring health protective working and living environment (Cancer Society of Finland, 2011; WHO/Health 2020, 2011). In case of lower income countries, strong orientation towards primary health care in performing programs of prevention and early detection of cancer, could be the best solution, as it has been proved that better primary care resources considerable contribute to reducing the adverse impact of social inequalities on health (Starfield, 2011). However, good primary care (practice) depends on good primary health care (system), that means that primary care is reflective of a specific health care system policy. This reasoning was in the background of the recent iniciative of the European Member States, to potentiate a wave of health reforms across Europe (WHO/Health 2020, 2011).

12. References

Ackerson, K. & Preston, S.D. (2009). A decision theory perspective on ehy women do or do not decide to have cancer screening: systematic review. *Journal of Advanced Nursing*, Vol. 65, No. 6, pp. (1130-1140).

Aebi, S., et al. On behalf of the ESMO Guidelines Workig Group. (2011). Primary breast cancer: ESMO clinical practice guidelines for diagnosis, treatment and follow-up. In: *Annals of Oncology*, Vol. 22, Suppl. 6, doi:10.1093/annonc/mdr371, October, 2011, available from: < www.esmo.org>

American Cancer Society. (2002). The American Cancer Society Guidelines on Nutrition and Physical Activity for Cancer Prevention. *CA-A Cancer Journal for Clinicians*, Vol. 52, No. 1, (March/April 2002), pp. (92-119).

American Cancer Society. (2011). Guidelines for Early Cancer Detection. In: *Cancer Facts & Figures (2011)*, October, 2011, available from: www.cancer.org

American Cancer Society. (2010). Guidelines for the Early Detection of Prostate Cancer: Update 2010. *CA: A Cancer Journal for Clinicians*, Vol. 60, (March/April) No. 2, pp. (70-98).

American Cancer Society. Written by Gould R.L. (1997/98). *Cancer and Genetics. A manual for Clinicians and Their Patients*, PRR, Inc., and the American Cancer Society, ISBN 9641823-6-x, New York.

Balmana, J., et al. (2010). Familial colorectal cancer risk: ESMO Clinical Practice Guidelines. *Annals of Oncology*, Vol. 21, Suppl. 5, pp. (v78-v81) doi:10.1093/annonc/mdq169

Balmana, J., et al. On behalf of the ESMO Guidelines Working Group. BRCA in breast cancer: ESMO Clinical Practice Guidelines. *Annals of Oncology*, Vol. 22, Suppl. 6, pp. (vi31-vi34).

Barlow, WE., et al. (2006). Prospective breast cancer risk prediction model for women undergoing screening mammography. *Journal of the National Cancer Institute*, Vol. 98, pp. (1204-1214).

Boccardo, E., Villa, L.L. (2011). Viral origins of human cancer. *Current Medicinal Chemistry*, Vol. 14, No. 24, pp. (2526-2539), ISSN: 0929-8673.

Boyle, P. (2003). Measuring progress against cancer in Europe: has the 15% decline targeted for 2000 come about? *Annals of Oncology*, Vol. 14, No. 8, pp. (1312-1325).

Brunekreef, B., et al. (2009). Effects of long-term exposure to traffic-related air pollution on respiratoy and cardiovascular mortality in the Netherlands: the NLCS-AIR study. *Research report (Health Effects Institute)*, Vol. 139, No. 5-71, pp. (73-89).

Butel, J.S. (1999). Viral carcinogenesis: revelation of molecular mechanisms and etiology of human disease. *Life Science & Medicine*, Vol. 21, No. 3, pp. (405-426).

Cancer Society of Finland. (2011). In: *Screening programme*, October 2011, available from: http://www.cancer.fi/syoparekisteri/en/mass-screening-registry/breast_cancer_screening/screening_programme/

Cancer screening in the EU - First Report. (2007). In: *Commission of the European Communities. Report on the implementation of the Council Recommendation on Cancer Screening - First Report*, October, 2011, available from:
< ec.europa.eu/health/archive/ph_determinants/.../cancer_screening.pdf>

Commission of the European Communities. (June, 2009). Communication from the Commission to The European Parlament, The Council, The European Economic and Social Committee and The Committee of the Regions on Action Against Cancer: European Partnership, In: *Commission of the European Communities, Brussels, 24.06.2009. COM (2009) 291/4*, June, 2011, available from:
< ec.europa.eu/anti.../EC-Antifraud-Strategy.pdf>

Daar, A.S, et al. (2007). Grand challenges in chronic non-communicable diseases. *Nature*, Vol. 450, No. 22, pp. (494-496).

Dempsey, A.F., et al. (2010). Examining future adolescent Human Papillomavirus vaccine uptake, with and without a school mandate. *Journal of Adolescent Health*, Vol. 47, pp. (242-248).

Derek, Y., et al. The global burden of chronic diseases. Overcoming impediments to prevention and control. *JAMA*, Vol. 291, No. 21, pp. (2616-2622).

Duffy, S.W., et al. Absolute numbers of lives saved and overdiagnosis in breast cancer screening, from a randomised trial and from the breast screening programme in England. *Journal of Medical Screening*, Vol. 17, pp. (25-30), DOI:10.1258/jms.2009.009094

Eberl, M.M., et al. BI-RADS classification for management of abnormal mammograms. *The Journal of the American Board of Family Medicine*, Vol. 19, No. 2, pp. (161-164).

Ebling, B., et al. (2007). Psycho-social aspects of measures aimed at decreasing prevalence of chronic diseases in the population of returnees in the Osijek Region, Croatia. *Collegium Antropologicum*, Vol. 31, No. 2, pp. (315-319).

El-Serag, H.B. (2011). Hepatocellular carcinoma. *The New England Journal of Medicine*, Vol. 365, pp. (1118-1127).

ESMO. (2010). European guidelines for quality assurance in cervical cancer screening. In: *ESMO. Scientific news 23.03.2010.*, September, 2011, available from: http://www.esmo.org/no_cache/view-news.html?tx_ttnews%5Btt_news%5D=809&tx_...

ESMO Guidelines Working Group. (2011). Prostate cancer: ESMO clinical practice guidelines for diagnosis, treatment and follow-up. In: *ESMO clinical practice guidelines: latest update titles*, October, 2011, available from:
<clinicalrecommendations@esmo.org>

European Commission. (June, 2011). Major and chronic diseases. Cancer, In: *Public health, European Commission*, June, 2011, available from:
<http://ec.europa.eu/health/major_chronic_diseases/diseases/cancer/index_en.htm>

Evans, J.P., et al. (2010). Preparing for a consumer-driven genomic age. *The New England Journal of Medicine*, Vol. 363, No. 12 (September, 2010), pp. (1099-1101).

Ferlay, J., et al. (2010). Cancer Incidence and Mortality Worldwode: IARC CancerBase No.10, In: *GLOBOCAN 2008, International Agency for Research on Cancer*, June, 2011, available from: <http://globocan.iarc.fr>

Flight, I.HK., et al. (8 Oct 2008). *Interventions for improving uptake of population-based screening for colorectal cancer using fecal occult blood testing*, John Willey 6 Sons, Retrieved from: <http://onlinelibrary.wiley.com/doi/10.1002/14651858.CD005035/full>

Harold, C.S. (2011). Better evidence about screening for lung cancer. *The New England Journal of Medicine*, Vol. 365, No. 5, pp. (455-457).

Hudson, K.L. (2011). Genomics, health care, and society. *The New England Journal of Medicine*, Vol. 365 (September, 2011), pp. (1033-1041).

Ioannidis, J.P. (2011). A roadmap for successful applications of clinical proteomics. *Proteomics - Clinical Applications*, Vol. 5, No. 5-6 (June, 2011), pp. (241-247).

Jellema, P., et al. (2010). Value of symptoms and additional diagnostic tests for colorectal cancer in primary care: systematic review and meta-analysis. In: *British Medical Journal*, September, 2011, available from: <http://www.bmj.com/content/340/bmj.c1269>

Jemal, A., et al. (2011). Global cancer statistics. In: *CA: A Cancer Journal for Clinicians*, DOI:10.3322/caac.20107, February, 2011, available from: <http://onlinelibrary.wiley.com/doi/10.3322/caac.20107/full>

Kovacs, A., et al. (2011). National cancer screening programme in Hungary. *Hrvatski časopis za javno zdravstvo [Croatian Journal for Public Health]*, Vol. 7, No. 27 (July, 2011), ISSN 1845-3082, September, 2011, available from: < http://www.hcjz.hr/clanak.php?id=14470>

Labianca, R., et al. (2010). Primary colon cancer: ESMO Clinical Practice Guidelines for diagnosis, adjuvant treatment and follow-up. *Annals of Oncology*, Vol. 21, Suppl. 5, pp. (v70-v77) doi:10.1093/annonc/mdq168

Lapaige, V. (2010). "Integrated knowledge translation" for globally oriented public health practitioners and scietnists: framing together a sustainable transfrontier knowledge translation vision. *Journal of Multidisciplinaey Healthcare*, Vol. 4, pp. (33-47).

Majnarić-Trtica, Lj., et al. (2008a): Is it time for a new approach in cardiovascular risk assessment? *Periodicum Biologorum*, Vol. 110, No. 1, pp. (45-50).

Majnarić-Trtica, Lj. et al. (2008b). Efforts in fighting against cancer in Croatia have to be focused on the primary health care. *Collegium Antropologicum*, Vol. 32, No. 3, pp. (709-724).

Majnarić-Trtica, Lj., et al. (2009). Trends and challenges in preventive medicine in European Union countries. Comment on the state in Croatia. *Periodicum Biologorum*, Vol. 111, No. 1, pp. (5-12), ISSN 0031-5362.

Mandelblatt, J.S., et al. (2011). To screen or not to screen women in their 40s for breast cancer: is personalized risk-based screening the answer? *Annals of Internal Medicine*, Vol. 155, No. 1 (July, 2011), pp. (58-60).

Masterson, S. & Owen, s. (2006). Mental health service user`s social and individual empowerment: Using theories of power to elucidate far-reaching strategies. *Journal of Mental Health*, Vol. 15, No. 1 (February, 2006), pp. (19-34).

McCorkie, R, et al. (2011). Self-management: enabling and empowering patients living with cancer as a chronic illness. *CA: A Cancer Journal for Clinicians*, Vol. 61, No. 1 (January/February, 2011), pp. (50-62).

Ministry of health and social welfare. (2006). *National Program for the Early Detection of Breast Cancer*, Croatian Oncological Society, Zagreb.

Ministry of health and social welfare. (2007). *National Program for the Early Detection of Colorectal Cancer*, Croatian Oncological Society, Zagreb.

NHS. UK. (2011). In: *The NHS cancer screening programmes*, October, 2011, available from: <http://www.cancerscreening.nhs.uk/>

O`Neill, SC., et al. (2008). Intentions to maintain adherence to mammography. *Journal of Womens Health*, Vol. 17, No. 7 (September, 2008), pp. (1133-1141).

Patridge, E.E. (2011). Elimination of cancer disparities via organizational transformation and communitydriven approaches. *CA: A Cancer Journal for Clinicians*, Vol. 61, No. 1 (January/February, 2011), pp. (5-7).

Pigeot, I., et al. (February, 2010). Primary prevention from the epidemiology perspective: three examples from the practice. In: *BMC Medical Research Methodology*, February, 2010, available from: <http://www.biomedcentral.com/1471-2288/10/10>

Pribić, S., et al. (2011). Colorectal cancer early detection program integrated in practice of family physicians. *Medicinski Glasnik Liječničke komore Zeničko-Dobojskog kantona*, Vol. 8, No.1, pp. (31-38).

Pribić, S., et al. (2010). Screening with mammography organized by family physicians teams: what have we learnt? *Collegium Antropologicum*, Vol. 34, No. 3, pp. (871-876).

Rosenbaum, A.M., et al. Clinical assesment incorporating a personal genome. *The Lancet*, Vol. 375, No. 9725 (May, 2010), pp. 1525-1535).

Samardžić, S., et al. (2007). A preliminary report of the Osijek-Baranja County, Croatia, on implementation of the National program for breast cancer screening. *Libri oncologici*, Vol. XXXV, No. 1-3, pp. (1-5).

Sandovici, I., et al. (2008). Dynamic epigenome: the impact of the environment on epigenetic regulation of gene expression and developmental programming. *Epigenetics*, Tost, J., pp. (343-370), Caister Academic Press, ISBN: 978-1-904455-23-3, Retrieved from: <http://www.horizonpress.com/epi>

Schiller, J.T., Lowy, D.R. (2010). Vaccines to prevent infections by oncoviruses. *Annual Review of Microbiology*, Vol. 64, pp. (23-41).

Schousboe, J.T., et al. (2011). Personalizing mammography by breast density and other risk factors for breast cancer: analysis of health benefits and cost-effectiveness. *Annual Internal Medicine*, Vo. 155, No. 1 (July, 2011), pp. (10-20).

Smith, R.A., et al. (2004). The randomized trials of breast cancer screening: what have we learned? *Radiologic clinics of North America*, Vol. 42, No. 5, (September, 2004), pp. (793-806).

Spitz, MR., et al. (2007). A risk model for prediction of lung cancer. *Journal of the National Cancer Institute*, Vol. 99, No. 9 (May, 2007), pp. (715-726).

Spitz, MR., et al. (2008). An expanded risk prediction model for lung cancer. *Cancer Prevention Research (Philadelphia)*, Vol. 1, No. 4 (September, 2008), pp. (250-254).

Starfield, B. (2011). Politics, primary healthcare and health: was Virchow right? *Journal of Epidemiology and Community Health*, Vol. 65, No. 8 (August, 2011), pp. (653-655).

Strnad, M. & Šogorić, S. Rano otkrivanje raka u Hrvatskoj [engl. Early detection of cancer in Croatia]. *Acta Medica Croatica*, Vol. 64, pp. (461-468).

Summerton, N. (2002). Cancer recognition and primary care. Editorial. *British Journal of General Practice*, (January, 2002), pp. (5-6).

Šamija, M., et al. (Eds.). (2007). *How to prevent and detect cancer early? Draft National Program*, Medicinska naklada, Zagreb.

The Sol Goldman Pancreatic Cancer Research Center. (2011). Are there screening tests available? In: *Johns Hopkins Medicine*, October, 2011, available from: <http://pathology.jhu.edu/pc/BasicScreening.php?area=ba>

UICC. (2007). Cancer control, In: *UICC Website: UICC Home*, February, 2007, available from: www.uicc.org.

UICC. (2006). World Cancer Declaration, In: *UICC World Cancer Congress*, April, 2007, available from: <www.worldcancercongress.org>

US National Cancer Institute. (June, 2010). Colorectal cancer risk assessment tool. In: *U.S. National Institutes of Health/National Cancer Institute*, September, 2011, available from: <http://www.cancer.gov/colorectalcancerrisk/>

US National Cancer Institute. (May, 2011). Cancer risk prediction resources. In: *U.S. National Institutes of Health/National Cancer Institute*, September, 2011, available from: <http://www.cancer.gov/colorectalcancerrisk/>

Venkat K.M. (2010). Global noncommunicable diseases - where worlds meet, In: *The New England Journal of Medicine*, September 17, 2010, available from: www.nejm.org

Wang, W., et al. (2007). PancPRO: risk assesment for individuals with a family history of pancreatic cancer. *Journal of Clinical Oncology*, Vol. 25, No. 11 (April, 2010), pp. (1417-1422).

Warner, E. (2011). Breast-cancer screening. *The New England Journal of Medicine*, Vol. 365, No. 11, pp. (1025-1032).

Weinberg, R.A. (1994). Oncogenes and tumor suppressor genes. In: *Chromosomes, genes and cancer*, American Cancer Society, pp. (160-171), J.B. Lippincott Company, New York

WHO/Cancer. (February, 2006). Cancer, In: Fact sheet N°297, March, 2007, available from: http://www. who.int/mediacentre/factsheets/fs297/en/print.html

WHO/Global health risks. (2009). Global health risks. mortality and burden of disease attributable to selected major risks. In: *WHO Library Cataloguing-in-Publication Data. Global health risks: mortality and burden of disease attributable to selected major risks*, May, 2011, available from: <www.who.int/healthinfo/global.../GlobalHealthRi>

WHO/Regional Office for Europe. (March, 2011). Developing the new European policy for health - Health 2020. In: First meeting of the European Health Policy Forum, May 2011, available from: www.euro.who.int/en/...health.../health-2020

3

Endometrial Cancer: Forecast

Fady S. Moiety and Amal Z. Azzam
University of Alexandria,
Egypt

1. Introduction

Abnormal uterine peri- and postmenopausal bleeding represent more than two thirds of the Gynecological consultations and the primary exclusion target off such presentations would be endometrial cancer.[1]Endometrial cancer is the most common malignancy of the female genital tract in the world and the seventh most common cause of death from cancer in women in western Europe.[2]The disease thus motivates the development of adequate prognostic determinants for more accurate triage of patients through various treatment modalities and to provide better insight into the cell biology of the disease.In recent years, certain factors have led to an increasing awareness of and emphasis on diagnosis and treatment of endometrial cancer. These factors include the declining incidence of cervical cancer and related deaths in the United States, prolonged life expectancy, postmenopausal use of hormone replacement therapy, and earlier diagnosis. Moreover, the availability of easily applied diagnostic tools and a clearer understanding of premalignant lesions of the endometrium have led to an increase in the number of women diagnosed with endometrial cancer.[3]Screening for the disease and thus its prediction is highly recommended, however , there is overlap between the terms prediction and forecast, as prediction implies that some outcome is expected, while a forecast may cover a range of possible outcomes.[4]

2. Risk factors[5]

- Associated with increased risk:

Obesity, Menopausal estrogen use, Diabetes mellitus, Nulliparity, Hypertension, Late menopause, Early menarche (<12 yrs), Polycystic ovarian syndrome, and Gall bladder disease.

- *Associated with decreased risk*: Smoking & Oral contraceptives

3. Presentation

Most cases of endometrial cancer are diagnosed in early stages because of abnormal uterine bleeding as the presenting symptom in 90% of the cases. (6) It is still debatable, which diagnostic tool is best performing for patients with postmenopausal bleeding. Hysteroscopy and/or hysteroscopic guided endometrial biopsies as well as endometrial sampling tools almost exclusively replaced the older modalities for investigating such cancer such as dilatation and curettage (D&C).[7]

The Pap test helped somehow in the past through incidental detection of some early cases with endometrial cancer, however, the test was proven to be of too low sensitivity and positive predictive value in terms of detecting both cervical and endometrial cancers.[8]It must be remembered that screening refers to the evaluation of the asymptomatic patient. When bleeding occurs, evaluation becomes diagnostic rather than screening. A history of bleeding or demonstrated radiographic evidence of endometrial pathology removes a patient from the realm of screening and demands investigation, i.e., an endometrial biopsy.[9]

While screening for endometrial cancer has been evaluated in prospective studies, the efficacy of endometrial screening has never been evaluated in a large prospective randomized controlled trial.Endometrial biopsy is easily performed as an office procedure and has good sensitivity, with the small number of false negatives most likely a result of sampling error. Transvaginal ultrasound (TVU) has also been used as a noninvasive screening test to evaluate the endometrium.[9]

4. Diagnosis

4.1. Screening of asymptomatic cases for early detection

High index of suspicion must be maintained if endometrial carcinoma will be diagnosed at an early stage. Postmenopausal bleeding should be taken to mean endometrial carcinoma until proved otherwise.[10]

1. **Transvaginal sonography (TVS):** is used to assess the endometrial thickness. This has been used as screening method combined with outpatient suction endometrial sampling (e.g. using a pipette). The cutoff thickness (myometrium to myometrium) expected in postmenopausal women, was once thought to be up to 8 mm.[11] If the endometrium is thickened or insufficient material is obtained by biopsy for diagnosis, then a more invasive procedure is required. This ideally comprises hysteroscopy accompanied or followed by a diagnostic curettage.[11]However, as yet, there is no agreed-upon criterion for endometrial thickness that has both a high sensitivity and specificity; a high rate of false-positive results is also a limiting factor.[12]

Previous meta-analyses on endometrial thickness measurement probably have overestimated its diagnostic accuracy in the detection of endometrial carcinoma. We advise the use of cutoff level of 3 mm for exclusion of endometrial carcinoma in women with postmenopausal bleeding.[13]

TVS has the added advantage of detecting any ovarian lesion and assessing the extent of myometrial involvement of endometrial cancer which can be achieved as efficient as Magnetic resonance imaging (MRI) utilization for the same purpose.[14]

2. Progesterone challenge test (PCT):

It is a reliable, non-invasive test to determine if estrogens, either endogenous or exogenous, are present in sufficient quantity to cause endometrial proliferation. Postmenopausal women with intact uterus should be given 100 milligrams of progesterone intramuscularly, if withdrawal bleeding follows, this indicates high endogenous estrogen priming the endometrium denoting a high risk patient. On the other hand, negative PCT i.e. no withdrawal bleeding, indicates low endogenous estrogen and consequently low risk patient. The test should be repeated on annual basis for those patients. [15]

3. Endometrial sampling:

Cytological study: to detect exfoliated malignant endometrial cells by a cervicovaginal smear or jet lavage aspiration. It, unfortunately, gives less reliable results than expected with a sensitivity of not more than 50%. (16)

Endometrial tissue biopsy: Accepted as a first step in evaluating a high-risk patient for endometrial carcinoma, with a diagnostic accuracy of 90 - 98%.

The endometrial tissue biopsy can be obtained using:

- Vacuum aspiration: using Carman's cannula which is 3-4mm diameter suction curette with 300-600 mm Hg negative pressure.
- Intrauterine brushing: using a metallic wire with nylon bristles rotated all over the uterine cavity.
- Novak or Randall curette: office procedure, without anesthesia, where scrapes are taken from each uterine wall and sent for histopathological examination.(17)

4.2. Diagnosis of symptomatic cases with postmenopausal uterine bleeding

Diagnostic curettage has been the standard means for the diagnosis of endometrial pathology. The naked-eye picture can be suggestive of malignancy if the curettings are profuse, in the form of cheesy lumps rather than strips and if they are dark in color. Failure of the uterine wall to "grate" with curetting is suggestive. However, histopathological confirmation should be-awaited.(18)

Fractional curettage (samples taken from the endocervix then from the endometrial cavity) can also be used to diagnose or exclude cervical involvement and thus for clinical staging. (19)

Hysteroscopy can be used in the diagnosis of endometrial carcinoma. Because 15-20% of the uterine cavity with possible malignant growth could be missed in conventional curettage, hysetroscope allows inspecting the endometrial cavity and indicating the site from which endometrial biopsy is to be taken under vision.(20)

4.3. Genetic analysis

Genetic testing for mutations in the mismatch repair genes is available, and if a pathogenic change is found within a family, predictive testing becomes available for unaffected family members to assess microsatellite instability, a feature of mismatch repair genes mutation.(21) On the other hand, immunohistochemical staining for p53 gene demonstrating overexpression of p53.(22)

Final diagnosis for pretreatment assessment and staging must entail:

Radiological imaging:

- Computer axial tomography (CT) scan with contrast can be helpful in pretreatment staging by identifying the depth of myometrial invasion, abdominal lymph node involvement, spread to pelvic and extra-pelvic organs, and ureteric invasion. (23)
- Magnetic resonance imaging (MRI) is a more advanced diagnostic tool in pretreatment staging with more accuracy and can detect much smaller tumor deposits and early cervical involvement.(24)

- Intravenous urography (IVU) to check for ureteric involvement.
- Plain X-ray chest to detect lung secondaries in advanced stage of the disease.
- Radioisotope scan to detect distant metastasis and bone deposits.
- Lymphangiography: for lymph node involvement for preoperative staging; it is now, however, replaced by CT scan.[18]
- Endoscopy: (in advanced cases)
- Cystoscopy: to detect bladder infiltration.
- Sigmoidoscopy: to check for rectal and sigmoid colon infiltration.[18]

4.4. Biochemical markers related to endometrial carcinoma:

Gynecologists happen to experience that patients with tumors that are identical in grade and stage often have significantly different clinical outcomes or responses to therapy. In order to identify an objective biological factor correlating with tumor aggressiveness, many tumor markers have been investigated. So far, **CA125** is one of the most reliable tumor marker for adenocarcinoma of the uterus and frequently used in a clinical setting. Elevated CA-125 levels have also been observed in serum, menstrual effluent, and the peritoneal fluid of women with endometrial carcinoma.[25]It can be assumed that if a patient with endometrial cancer had an elevated preoperative CA 125, it would probably be a cancer with poor prognosis. Thus, CA 125 is considered a positive marker in these cases and its high production is associated with increased metastatic potential. In addition, CA 125 levels were found to be independent risk factor for pelvic lymph node metastasis.[26, 27]

Not only in the sera of patients with endometrial carcinoma, do CA 125 levels rise significantly, but also in their tissues. Cancer tissues contain CA 125 and the percentage of positive CA 125 tissue staining is significantly higher than that of elevated CA 125 serum levels. An increase in serum CA125 after operation predicted the possibility of recurrence. [28, 29]

The potent cytokine; tumor necrosis factor alpha **(TNF-α)** was first identified to be synthesized and secreted by the human endometrium. The endometrial epithelial cells are a major source of TNF-α. TNF-α may be useful in the discrimination of malignant from benign gynecological diseases and in monitoring tumor activity in patients early in the malignancy process. [30, 31, 32]

Tumor necrosis factor alpha (TNF α) concentration was determined by a solid phase immunoradiometric assay. The rate of abnormally high values of serum TNF α increased with advancing stage of the disease. On the other hand, serum TNF α level in cases of endometrial hyperplasia was significantly lower than in healthy individuals. It seems that the rise of serum TNF α in cases of endometrial carcinoma represents a possible mechanism of immune surveillance. It is thus suggested that serum TNF α estimations for the differential diagnosis of benign and malignant lesions of the endometrium in women with postmenopausal bleeding could be beneficial. [33]

4.5. Prognostic factors[19]

Multiple factors have been identified which significantly influence the prognosis in endometrial carcinoma; some of these factors are interdependent:

Prognostic factors in endometrial carcinoma:

1. Age and body morphology.
2. Stage.
3. Histopathologic type.
4. Histologic differentiation.
5. Depth of myometrial invasion.
6. Lymph node involvement.
7. Peritoneal cytology.
8. Steroid receptor status
9. DNA ploidy.
10. Molecular indices.

1. Age and body morphology:

Older patients do worse. Obese patients do better than lean ones. It seems that the obese, hyperlipidemic women, with evidence of unopposed estrogen exposure like anovulatory uterine bleeding, infertility, late menopause, and hyperplasia of ovarian stroma tend to have more differentiated endometrial carcinoma with better prognosis.

2. Stage:

Involvement of the cervix definitely worsens the prognosis; cervical stromal invasion is worse than involvement of the endocervix only. The overall survival rate for endometrial cancer is high as there is a preponderance of women diagnosed with stage I disease.

3. Histological type:

The rare tumor types of endometrial carcinoma like serous papillary, clear cell and squamous carcinoma have a definitely poorer prognosis than usual enometrioid adenocarcinoma. The frequent presence of squamous metaplasia not showing malignant feature i.e. adenoacanthoma, does not change the prognosis.

4. Histological differentiation: Tumor grade:

As the tumor gets less differentiated, the risk of deep myometrial invasion increases. Within each stage the prognosis is therefore, influenced by the tumor grade.

5. Depth of myometrial invasion:

Deep invasion is associated with higher rates of lymph node involvement and is usually associated with lesser degrees of differentiation. Reaching the serosa will shift the disease to stage III and is associated with poor prognosis.

6. Lymph node involvement:

There is a good deal of correlation between lymph node involvement and other prognostic factors. In stage I disease, the incidence of pelvic lymph node involvement is about 10 % and the 5-years survival in these subset is only 30% as compared with more than 70% for the whole of stage I cases. [34]

7. Peritoneal cytology:

Obtaining peritoneal washings for cytology examination is an easy procedure for assessment of prognosis. However, its value independent of other prognostic indicators is not fully established. [35]

8. Hormone (steroid) receptor status:

Estrogen receptor and progesterone receptor levels have been shown to be prognostic indicators for endometrial cancers independent of grade. Patients with tumors positive for one or both receptors have longer survival than patients whose carcinomas lack the corresponding receptors. Even patients with metastasis have an improved prognosis with receptor positive tumors. Progesterone receptor levels appear to be stronger predictors of survival than estrogen receptor levels, and the higher the absolute level of the receptor, the better the prognosis. [36]

9. DNA ploidy and proliferative index:

Flow cytometry has been used in assessment of the ploidy of the tumor. This determines cellular nuclear DNA content and measures the fraction of the tumor cells in proliferative phase (S- phase). Flow cytometry will determine DNA histogram, which reflects the cell cycle phase. G0 and G1 cells contain diploid nuclear DNA content. In a well-differentiated tumor, a smaller number of cells enter the S-phase and begin DNA replication (S-phase fraction). DNA ploidy can be denoted as DNA index (DI), which is the numerical ratio of DNA content of the tumor cells to the DNA content of G0/G1 peak of normal control population. A diploid tumor has a DI range of 0.95 % to 1.1 and a tetraploid tumor has a DI range of 1.9 to 2%; peaks outside these ranges e.g. 1.5 or 2.6 are defined as aneuploid. Most endometrial cancers are diploid but aneuploidy indicates advanced disease and a poor prognosis. A raised fraction of cells in the S-phase (with DI around 2) also indicates a poor prognosis.

10. Genetic and molecular markers:

Analysis of the mutations in mismatch repair (MMR) genes can be achieved through studying blood samples or tumor blocks to assess microsatellite instability, a feature of mismatch repair gene mutations. These mutations have been reported in 10% to 20% of endometrial adenocarcinomas. Alteration of the tumor suppressor gene p53 has also been demonstrated in about 20% of endometrial carcinomas and has been associated with papillary serous cell type, advanced stage and poor prognosis. [37,38]

In summary, endometrial cancer screening, and thus its outcome prediction (forecast) seem to be achievable in a more variety of ways than any other female genital malignancy. Early detection is definitely the first step to attain a complete cure. The management options for endometrial cancer, and thus the survival rate from the disease would depend largely on early detection modalities mentioned above. The following are some recommendations from the American cancer Society (ACS) for early detection of the disease based on patients' characteristics.(9)*Recommendations for Women at Average Risk:* There is no indication that screening for endometrial cancer is warranted for women who have no identified risk factors.[39]

Recommendations for Women at Increased Risk: There is no indication that screening for endometrial cancer should be recommended for women at increased risk for endometrial cancer because of history of unopposed estrogen therapy, late menopause, tamoxifen therapy, nulliparity, infertility or failure to ovulate, obesity, diabetes, or hypertension.(39)

Recommendations for Women at High Risk: The American Cancer Society recommends that annual screening for endometrial cancer with endometrial biopsy should be offered by age 35 for women with or at risk for hereditary nonpolyposis colorectal cancer (HNPCC). Women in this high-risk group should be informed about the risks and symptoms of endometrial cancer, and should be informed about potential benefits, risks, and limitations of testing for early endometrial cancer detection.

5. References

[1] Mencaglia L. Hysteroscopy and adenocarcinoma. ObstetGynecolClin North Am 1995;22: 573–579.

[2] Colombo N, Preti E, Landoni F, Carinelli S, Colombo A, Marini C, Sessa C; ESMO Guidelines Working Group.Endometrial cancer: ESMO Clinical Practice Guidelines for diagnosis, treatment and follow-up. Ann Oncol. 2011 Sep;22Suppl 6:vi35-9.

[3] Laurin JR. Uterine cancer In: Berek JS, Rinehart RD, Hillard PA, and Adashi EY (eds.) Novak's Gynecology. 13th edition. Philadelphia: Lippincott Williams & Wilkins publications, 2002, (30): 1150-62.

[4] http://en.wikipedia.org/wiki/Prediction

[5] Piver MS, and Marchetti DL. Endometrial carcinoma In: Piver MS (ed.) Gynecologic oncology. London: Chapman & Hall publications 1998;(7): 87-8.

[6] Soeters R, Denny LA. Cancer of the uterus In: Lawton F, Friedlander M, and Thomas G. (eds): Essentials of gynecologic cancer. London: Chapman & Hall publications, 1998; (9):158-60.

[7] Cooper JM, Erickson ML. Endometrial sampling techniques in the diagnosis of abnormal uterine bleeding.*ObstetGynecolClin North Am* 2000; *27:* 235–244.

[8] Walker JL, Nunez ER. Endometrial cancer, in KramerBS, GohaganJK, ProrokPC (eds): Cancer Screening: Theory And Practice. New York, Marcel Dekker, Inc., 1999, pp 531–566.

[9] Smith RA, von Eschenbach AC, Wender R, Levin B, Byers T, Rothenberger D, Brooks D, Creasman W, Cohen C, Runowicz C, Saslow D, Cokkinides V, Eyre H; ACS Prostate Cancer Advisory Committee, ACS Colorectal Cancer Advisory Committee, ACS Endometrial Cancer Advisory Committee. American Cancer Society guidelines for the early detection of cancer: update of early detection guidelines for prostate, colorectal, and endometrial cancers. Also: update 2001--testing for early lung cancer detection. CA Cancer J Clin. 2001 Jan-Feb;51(1):38-75; quiz 77-80. Erratum in: CA Cancer J Clin 2001 May-Jun;51(3):150.

[10] Blake P., Lambert H., and Crawford R. Gynecological oncology, a guide to clinical management. Oxford medical publications 1998; (4):76-83.

[11] Gull B, Karlsson B, Milsom I, and Granberg S. Can ultrasound replace dilation and curettage? A longitudinal evaluation of postmenopausal bleeding and transvaginal sonographic measurement of the endometrium as predictors of endometrial cancer. Int J Cancer 2001; 94(6): 795-9.

[12] Weigel M, Friese K, Strittmater HJ, Melchert F. Measuring the thickness - is that all we have to do for sonographic assessment of endometrium in postmenopausal women? *Ultrasound ObstetGynecol*1995; 6: 97–102

[13] Timmermans A, Opmeer BC, Khan KS, Bachmann LM, Epstein E, Clark TJ, Gupta JK, Bakour SH, van den Bosch T, van Doorn HC, Cameron ST, Giusa MG, Dessole S, Dijkhuizen FP, TerRiet G, Mol BW. Endometrial thickness measurement for detecting endometrial cancer in women with postmenopausal bleeding: a systematic review and meta-analysis. Obstet Gynecol. 2010 Jul;116(1):160-7.

[14] Sawicki W, Spiewankiewicz B, Stelmachow J, and Cendrowski K. The value of ultrasonography in preoperative assessment of selected prognostic factors in endometrial cancer. Eur J GynaecolOncol. 2003;24(3-4):293-8.

[15] Gambrell RD Jr. Massey FM. Castaneda TA, Ugenas AJ, Ricci CA, and Wright JM. Use of the progesterone challenge test to reduce the risk of endometrial cancer. Obstetrics and Gynecology 1980; 55: 732-8.

[16] Zucker PK, Kasdon EJ, and Feldstein ML. The validity of PAP smear parameters as predictors of endometrial pathology in menopausal women. Cancer 1985; 56: 2256-63.

[17] Greenwood SM, and Wright DJ. Evaluation of the office endometrial biopy in the detection of endometrial carcinoma and atypical hyperplasia. Cancer 1979; 43:1474-8.

[18] Anderson B. Diagnosis of endometrial cancer In: Creasman WT (ed): Clinics In Obstetrics And Gynecology- Endometrial Cancer. London: W.B Saunders Company, 1986; Vol 13, (5): 739-47.

[19] Bhatla N. Tumors of the corpus uteri. In: Bhatla N. (ed.)Jeffcoate's Principles Of Gynecology. 5th edition. London: Arnold publications, 2001 (26): 466-71.

[20] Valle RF. Hysteroscopic evaluation of patients with abnormal uterine bleeding. Surgery, Gynecology and Obstetrics 1981; 15:521-6.

[21] Lalloo F, and Evans G. Molecular genetics and endometrial cancer. Best Pract Res ClinObstetGynaecol 2001; 15(3): 355-63.

[22] Ohkouchi T, Sakuragi N, Watari H, Nomura E, Todo Y, Yamada H, and Fujimoto S. Prognostic significance of Bcl-2, p53 overexpression, and lymph node metastasis in surgically staged endometrial carcinoma Am J ObstetGynecol 2002(187): 15-7.

[23] Chen SS, Kumari S, and Lee L. contribution of abdominal computed tomography (CT) in the management of Gynecologic cancer: correlated study of CT image and gross surgical pathology. GynecolOncol 1980; 10:162-72.

[24] Haricak H, Lacey C, and Schriock E. Gynecologic masses: value of magnetic resonance imging. Am J ObstetGynecol 1985; 153:31-7.

[25] Numa F, Umayahara K, Suehiro Y, Suminami Y, Oga A, Sasaki K, and Kato H. New molecular tumor markers for endometrial cancer.Hum Cell - 2001; 14(4): 272-4.

[26] Kukura V, Zovko G, Ciglar S, Markulin-Grgic L, Santek F, Podgajski M, and Duic Z. Serum CA-125 tumor marker in endometrial adenocarcinoma. Eur J GynaecolOncol. 2003; 24(2):151-3.

[27] Todo Y, Sakuragi N, Nishida R, Yamada T, Ebina Y, Yamamoto R, and Fujimoto S. Combined use of magnetic resonance imaging, CA 125 assay, histologic type, and histologic grade in the prediction of lymph node metastasis in endometrial carcinoma. Am J Obstet Gynecol. 2003 ;189(2):567.

[28] Ginath S, Menczer J, Fintsi Y, Ben-Shem E, Glezerman M, and Avinoach I. Tissue and serum CA125 expression in endometrial cancer..Int J Gynecol Cancer. 2002;12(4): 372-5.

[29] Xie Z, Zhang J, and Tan A. Relationship between serum CA125 level and prognosis in the patients with uterine endometrial carcinoma. Zhonghua Yi XueZaZhi. 2001 10;81(23):1456-7.

[30] Tabibzadeh, S. Ubiquitous expression of TNF-alpha/Cachectin in human endometrium. Am. J. Rep. Immunol. 1991 : 26, 1–5.

[31] Tabibzadeh, S. Signals and molecular pathways involved in apoptosis with special emphasis on human endometrium. Hum. Reprod. Update. 1995: 1, 303–23.

[32] Sarandakou A, Phocas I, Sikiotis K, Rizos D, Botsis D, Kalambokis K, Trakakis E, and Chryssikopoulos A. Cytokines in gynecological cancer. Anticancer Res. 1997; 17(5B): 3835-9.

[33] ShaarawyM, and Abdel-Aziz O. Serum tumor necrosis factor alpha levels in benign and malignant lesions of the endometrium in postmenopausal women. A preliminary study. ActaOncol. 1992;31(4):417-20.

[34] Grigsby PW. Stage II carcinoma of the endometrium: Results of therapy and prognostic factors. Int J. Radiat. Oncol. Biol. Phys, 1985; 11:1915.

[35] Yazigi R, Piver MS, and Blumenson L. Malignant peritoneal cytology as a prognostic indicator on stage I endometrial cancer. Obstet Gynecol. 1983; 62:359.

[36] BozdoLan O, Atasoy P, Erekul S, BozdoLan N, and Bayram M. Apoptosis-related proteins and steroid hormone receptors in normal, hyperplastic, and neoplastic endometrium. Int J Gynecol 2002;21(4):375-82.

[37] Maeda K, Tsuda H, Hashiguchi Y, Yamamoto K, Inoue T, and Ishiko O. Relationship between p53 pathway and estrogen receptor status in endometrioid-type endometrial cancer. Hum Pathol 2002; 33(4):386-91.

[38] Ohkouchi T, Sakuragi N, and Watari H. Prognostic significance of Bcl-2, p53 overexpression, and lymph node metastasis in surgically staged endometrial carcinoma. Am J ObstetGynecolVol 187 (2) 2002:42-5.

[39] Kim YB, Ghosh K, Ainbinder S, Berek JS. Diagnostic and therapeutic advances in gynecologic oncology: screening for gynecologic cancer. Cancer Treat Res 1998; 95: 253-276.

4

Long-Term Venous Access in Oncology: Chemotherapy Strategies, Prevention and Treatment of Complications

Rykov Maxim and Buydenok Yury
Institute of Pediatric Oncology and Hematology, N. N. Blokhin Cancer Research Center, Moscow, Russia

1. Introduction

Increasing the effectiveness of current chemotherapy strategies requires a higher dosage, the greater duration of treatment, multiple chemotherapy cycles, and strong adherence to recommended interval lengths between cycles. Anticancer drug administration (usually intravenously) may result in vessel wall irritation, phlebitis/phlebothrombosis, and tissue necrosis due to accidental drug extravasation. The small diameter of a peripheral vein, low blood flow velocity, easy bacterial invasion due to the proximity of the blood vessel to the contaminated skin frequently and quickly result in the aforementioned complications which render peripheral veins impossible to use as a venous access. A central venous access allows physicians to avoid most of these problems. However, its use may also lead to complications including infection, thrombosis and aeroembolism. Apart from that, multiple blood vessel punctures and a central vein catheterization for diagnostic tests, chemotherapy, maintenance treatment, and intravenous feeding have a negative effect on the quality of life. It should also be kept in mind that in pediatrics such an intrusive diagnostic method is done under general anesthesia, which is hazardous, by itself. Since a cancer treatment lasts for many months and even years, patients with traditional subclavian catheters face a significant decrease in quality of life, and experience difficulties in providing personal hygiene. This results in serious complications, the most dangerous of them being a catheter-related infection and a catheter sepsis. They are often caused by a slight shift in a catheter position, which allows the pus from the puncture wound to enter the patient's bloodstream along the outer wall of the catheter. Children may quite frequently put themselves in danger by removing an external catheter while receiving chemotherapy. It is especially dangerous if it occurs within the period of pancytopenia when the low blood count eliminates the option of a subclavian catheter, and thus an adjunctive therapy has to be given via a peripheral venous access. All the abovementioned issues may postpone the next treatment stage and ultimately have a negative effect on the whole treatment strategy and decrease its effectiveness.

Thus, the use of a totally implantable venous access system (portacath) is preferable. It is unaffected by external factors when it is not used for infusion, it is comfortable, provides a high quality of life, and is installed once lasting for the whole therapy period.

2. Materials and methods

Since 2000, more than 1500 oncological patients (aged from 6 months to 87 years) of the N.N. Blokhin Cancer Research Center have had a totally implantable venous access system installed subcutaneously.

A port is a reservoir compartment made of metal (titanium) or plastic (polysulphone). The base of a port has a device securing it in a fixed position, while the upper part contains a silicone septum, which can be punctured multiple times with a special needle for drawing blood, drug administration, and flushing the device. A catheter is attached to the side of the port with the distal end of the former located in the central vein. A dual chamber port is used when the current treatment strategies require simultaneous administration of incompatible drugs.

A port implantation requires a sterile environment, and that is why it is performed in an operating room. It is done under local anesthesia in adults and general anesthesia in children. The port can also be used for preoperative management.

Successful venous access system implantation requires an ultrasound-guided transcutaneous catheterization of the superior vena cava via an external jugular, internal jugular or subclavian vein (using a subclavicular or supraclavicular approach). An access to the superior vena cava via an internal jugular or subclavian vein (with a supraclavicular approach) is preferred to an easier traditional subclavicular approach to the subclavian vein. The latter option is undesirable, for the catheter may get lodged between the first rib and the clavicle and eventually rupture leading to drug extravasation. Another problem is connected with possibility that the catheter can be torn off.

It should be noted that an adjacent artery injury may occur during venipuncture, in which case pulsing bright red blood enters the vein under great pressure resulting in a hematoma formation and its infection. This decreases the odds of success when attempting to gain a venous access from the chosen venipuncture site.

The central vein catheterization in the neck area may also lead to an accidental puncture and trauma of thoracic duct, nerve plexus, phrenic, vagus and recurrent nerve, esophagus, larynx and trachea. Gaining a central venous access in the clavicle area bears the risk of an accidental puncture and trauma of subclavian artery, pleural cavity, lung and brachial plexus. In case of thoracic duct puncture (a rare complication of attempting to gain left-sided venous access) the catheter gets filled with milk colored fluid - lymph. The needle should be instantly removed and adequate pressure applied for 5 - 10 minutes to avoid formation of a hematoma. The subsequent venous access has to be located on the other side or as far as possible from the previous one.

A nerve plexus trauma is characterized by neurological symptoms and acute pain reminiscent of an electric shock. This complication also requires immediate needle withdrawal.

In case of an airway puncture and a lung tissue trauma, air appears in the syringe. However, this may be also due to loose connection of the syringe with the needle. As a result crepitation can be heard upon neck and thorax palpation and the patient complains of shortness of breath and chest pain caused by an increasing pneumothorax. In some patients, pneumothorax is asymptomatic and is diagnosed by thorough auscultation and X-ray examination. The outcome depends on the rate of the pneumothorax progression, its severity and swift conversion of a closed pneumothorax to an open one by means of thoracostomy. Each central vein catheterization should be followed by chest x-ray. This allows to verify the position of the catheter and to assess the cardiovascular system.

In order to avoid the aforementioned complications a venipuncture should be performed under ultrasound control.

Successful use of an implantable venous access system is only possible when the distal end of the catheter is situated in the superior vena cava above its opening into the right atrium. The position of the catheter in the superior vena cava is most accurately determined by X-ray visualization in a cath lab or general operating room equipped with an electron-optical image intensifier. These methods are preferable in pediatric oncology for small vein diameter makes it quite hard to drive the guidewire precisely into the superior vena cava and avoid its entry into cervical veins. Accurate catheter position monitoring can also be achieved with the help of an endocardial electrogram. However, we recommend against using this method in children.

Following the catheter implantation a 2 - 4 cm incision is done below the puncture site. The length of the incision depends on the port chamber size. A special subcutaneous recess (or pocket) is made below the incision and a subcutaneous tunnel is formed using a tunneler, which is included in the implantable port kit. Afterwards the catheter is led through the subcutaneous tunnel into the port chamber with the help of a tunneler. Then the port chamber is inserted into the subcutaneous recess and fixed with interrupted sutures to the adjacent tissues and the incision is closed layer by layer. Throughout the implantation drawing some blood from the catheter or the port with a Huber needle constantly checks procedure the position of the catheter and the port. The port is ready for the infusion several hours after implantation.

The steps of the surgery are listed below:

1. Internal jugular vein ultrasound mapping;
2. Internal jugular vein puncture;
3. Guidewire insertion with radioscopic monitoring and needle removal;
4. Dilator (bougie) insertion over the guidewire;
5. Guidewire removal from the catheter and clamping of the latter to avoid hemorrhage and aeroembolism;
6. Catheter insertion into the dilator filled with normal saline;
7. Blood withdrawal and immediate catheter flushing for prevention of thrombosis;
8. Skin incision in the subclavian area below the puncture site;
9. Subcutaneous pocket formation below the incision;
10. Dilator removal (splitting);
11. Subcutaneous tunnel formation which links the skin pocket to the puncture site;
12. Catheter tunneling from the puncture site to the skin pocket and positioning in the superior vena cava under X-ray monitoring;
13. Additional blood withdrawal and catheter flushing;
14. Ligature appliance in the skin pocket and port chamber fixation;
15. Port chamber and catheter connection, and fixing it in place with a special lock;
16. Port insertion into the skin pocket and ligation;
17. Layer by layer incision closure above the port;
18. Blood withdrawal from the port chamber with a Huber needle and thorough flushing with normal saline followed by a heparin lock introduction.

The port puncture should only be done with a special Huber needle whose tip is designed to rule out the possibility of the silicon septum damage. The retrograde blood flow from the venous port upon slight aspiration is indicative of the proper infusion system functioning. Unlike regular needles, a Huber needle does not cut the silicone port septum, "spreading" it instead and keeping the system airtight for several years. The port puncture is a simple procedure, while the infusion system management requires trained staff. The port puncture can be repeated up to 2000 times provided it is performed with Huber needles which in theory allow using the system weekly for 40 years.

A visual check is needed prior to the needle insertion. If no signs of inflammation are present, the exact location of the septum is determined by palpation. Afterward while the port is kept in place between the index finger and the thumb, the needle is inserted vertically through the skin and the septum until it reaches the posterior wall of the port chamber. When accessing the port, the sterility should be ensured that implies the use of sterile gloves when performing the puncture. Modern antiseptics should be used for skin disinfection above the port and the puncture needle should be covered with disposable sterile dressing. Long presence of bacterial growth facilitating media (blood, proteins, amino acids, carbohydrates) in the port chamber and use of solutions from previously opened bottles (this especially concerns heparin) should be avoided. If needle insertion is successful, blood is drawn into the syringe upon careful aspiration. The blood (1 - 2 ml) should be disposed of and the port should be immediately flushed with 20.0 ml of normal saline. 10 ml or bigger syringes are needed in order to prevent catheter disconnection from the port chamber by excessive pressure. An incorrect insertion of the needle into the port may lead to extravasation and a fluid bleb formation in the port area.

After the infusion is complete and the needle is removed the patient can resume his normal life, bathe and even go swimming.

There are three main complications, which can pose a problem for prolonged central venous access use - thrombophlebitis at the site of the central venous catheter implantation, catheter thrombosis, and infusion system contamination with consequent infection.

The first complication is characterized by an edema, cyanosis and sometimes the hyperthermia of the upper limb and neck at the site of the venous access. Thrombophlebitis spread and progression rate is monitored with ultrasound. Chest X-ray and bacteriological study of the intravenous fluid in the catheter and port are highly recommended. The port should be removed if clinical situation allows it. In some cases it can be left in place provided the anticoagulant therapy is given promptly and contraindications are absent.

Catheter thrombosis is most likely to occur due to the venous access system mismanagement when the medical staff fails to flush the port after blood withdrawal or infusion. The preferred drug for the port flushing is urokinase - a fibrinolytic agent that activates glu-plasminogen and lys-plasminogen and converts them into plasmin, which causes enzymatic breakdown of fibrin. Fibrin mesh breakdown leads to clot disintegration and fragmentation. Clot fragments are then carried off with the blood flow or dissolved in situ. 2 - 2.5 ml of urokinase should be introduced into the system with exposure time of 15 minutes, followed by its aspiration from the portacath.

The infusion system contamination is a very dangerous condition that poses a threat of generalized sepsis. The first and rather reliable sign of the portacath contamination is high fever and algor developing 30 minutes after the introduction of normal saline into the port.

Contamination usually occurs in the infusion system inner environment and the implantation site may show no local signs even if the portacath is left unused. However, inflammation signs, often accompanied by thrombophlebitis, may be present at the site of the venous access system. The diagnosis can be verified with a bacteriological study of the fluid present in the infusion system and if it is, the venous access system has to be removed. The main cause of infusion system contamination is the medical staff's failure to comply with basic rules of infection prevention, which include washing hands and using sterile gloves and masks. One of the leading causes of contamination is multiple normal saline withdrawal from one 400 ml bottle (5 - 10 ml of normal saline are mixed with a 25000 IU heparin solution to prepare the infusion system lock). The 400 ml bottle is not changed within a shift and is stored under inadequate conditions. As a result, the absence of pharmaceutical forms for central and peripheral venous catheter flushing leads to severe complications and high costs of long-term treatment of serious catheter-associated infections. In this regard, TauroPharm's novel drug - TauroLock - is of great interest to physicians. The drug is specifically designed for flushing and locking of catheters, ports, and other long-term vascular access systems in cancer patients, patients undergoing surgery, patients with cancer, kidney failure, etc. TauroLock contains sodium citrate and taurolidine. The former is an anticoagulant and the latter is a new antimicrobial agent with a high antibacterial, antiviral and antifungal activity. The drug is so efficient in the catheter infection prophylaxis and treatment in cancer patients, that infusion system removal is not required.

According to several studies, the leading cause of catheter-associated infection in patients with a totally implantable venous access system is S. epidermidis, which is known to colonize mucous membranes and skin and contaminate the port chamber during the needle entry despite adherence to the rules of infection prevention. The authors use EMLA cream containing lidocaine and prilocaine to provide the topical anesthesia prior to a Huber needle insertion into the port chamber. The cream also has antibacterial properties provided that the exposition is 40 - 60 minutes.

3. Results

The postoperative period was uneventful with only one case of the skin pocket infection successfully treated with antibiotics. All the patients feel comfortable with having subcutaneous venous access ports. Children have no fear of catheterization prior to yet another chemotherapy cycle and are not afraid of Huber needle insertion owing to the use of the anesthetizing cream. Since the implantation, all the systems have been functioning adequately. Six patients developed the port system thrombosis, which was efficiently coped with by means of urokinase introduction into the infusion system with a 15-minute exposition. No cases of a catheter-associated infection were reported.

We use two types of solutions for port system locking between infusions - a 100 IU/ml heparin solution and Taurolock (TauroPharm, Germany), a drug specifically designed to be used as an infusion system lock.

4. Conclusion

The implantable venous port system use in cancer treatment allows physicians to reduce the number of invasive procedures, less often resort to general anesthesia, and significantly increase the patients' quality of life by offering the possibility to return to their normal lives, i.e. to take up sports (including aquatics) and follow regular hygiene procedures. Apart from that, the port is almost unnoticeable under the skin. In the case of external venous access systems, a chemotherapy cycle could be delayed if it was impossible to gain venous access for some reason (inadequate blood count or organ failure that did not allow for general anesthesia). With the introduction of implantable port systems each chemotherapy cycle can be started on time provided that there are no other counterindications.

5. References

[1] Berezhanski B. V. Optimizatsiya farmakoterapii i profilaktiki infektsij svyazannih s tsentralnim venosnim kateterom v otdelenijah reanimatsii i intensivnoj terapii. Published summary of a thesis (candidate of Medical Science) Smolensk, 2008. p. 22. (In Russian)

[2] Gualtieri E, Deppe SA, Sipperly ME, Thompson DR. Subclavian venous catheterization: greater success rate for less experienced operators using ultrasound guidance. Vestnik Intensivnoy Terapii, 2006, №4. p 24-30

[3] Egiev V. N, Shetinin V. V., Trofimenko Y. G., Polnostju implantiruemie sistemi v meditsine. Medpraktika-M, Moscow, 2004, p 60. (In Russian)

[4] Noble V. E., Nelson B., Sutingco A. N. Manual of Emergency and Critical Care Ultrasound. Meditsinskaya literatura, 2009, p 227.

[5] Suhorukov V.P., Berdikyan A. S., Epshtein S. L. Punktsiya i kateterizatsiya ven. Traditsionnie i novie tehnologii. Posobie dlya vrachey, Sankt-Peterburgskoye meditsinskoye izdatelstvo, 2001, p 55. (In Russian)

[6] Rudolph R., Larson D.L. // Journal Clin. Oncol. — 1987. - Vol. 5. - P. 1116-1126.

[7] Fuchs R, Leimer L, Koch G, Westerhausen M. Klinische Erfahrungen mit bakteriell kontaminierten Port-a-Cath Systemen bei Tumorpatienten. Dtsch Med Wochenschr 1987;112:1615–8.

[8] Gowardman JR, Montgomery C, Thirlwell S, et al. Central venous catheter-related bloodstream infections: an analysis of incidence and risk factors in a cohort of 400 patients. Intensive Care Med 1998;24:1034–9.

[9] Timsit JF, Farkas JCH, Boyer JM, et al. Central vein catheter-related thrombosis in intensive care patients: incidence, risk factors, and relationship with catheter-related sepsis. Chest 1998;114:207–13.

[10] Daschner FD. The transmission of infection in hospitals by staff carriers, methods of prevention and control. Infect Control 1985;6:97–8.

[11] Darouiche RO, Raad II, Heard SO, et al., Catheter Study Group. A comparison of two antimicrobial-impregnated central venous catheters. N Engl J Med 1999;340:1–8.

[12] Erb F, Imbenotte M, Huveene J. Structural investigation of a new organic antimicrobial: taurolidine analytical study and application to identification and quantitation in biological fluids. Eur J Drug Metab Pharmacokinet 1983;8:163–73.

[13] Gorman SP, McCafferty DF, Woolfson AD, Jones DS. Reduced adherence of micro-organisms to human mucosal epithelial cells following treatment with Taurolin®, a novel antimicrobial agent. J Appl Bacteriol 1987;62:315–20.

[14] Monson JR, Ramsey PS, Donohue JH. Taurolidine inhibits tumour necrosis factor (TNF) toxicity—new evidence of TNF and endotoxin synergy. Eur J Surg Oncol 1993;19:226–31.

[15] Leithauser ML, Rob PM, Sack K. Pentoxifylline, cyclosporine A and taurolidine inhibit endotoxin-stimulated tumour necrosis factor-alpha production in rat mesangial cell cultures. Exp Nephrol 1997;5:100–4.

5

Early Detection and Prevention of Breast Cancer: The Increasing Importance of Midwives in the Future

Andrej Plesničar[1], Klaudia Urbančič[1], Suzana Mlinar[1], Božo Kralj[2], Viljem Kovač[3] and Blanka Kores Plesničar[4]
[1]*University of Ljubljana, Faculty of Health Sciences, Ljubljana*
[2]*University of Ljubljana, Faculty of Medicine, Ljubljana*
[3]*Institute of Oncology, Ljubljana*
[4]*University of Maribor, Faculty of Medicine, Maribor*
Slovenia

1. Introduction

Breast cancer (BC) is the most common type of cancer and cause of death from cancer in women in the Republic of Slovenia. As in the majority of other economically and industrially developed countries, the incidence rate of BC is increasing in Slovenia and has reached 111.8 cases per 100,000 women in 2008. The incidence rate of BC has thus shown more than a fivefold increase in the period from 1950 to 2008 and BC was diagnosed in 1,147 women in 2008 (Cancer Registry of Republic of Slovenia, 2010). Similar increases in the incidence rates of BC have in the last decades also been observed in a number of other economically and industrially developed countries with aging female population (Curado et al (Eds.), 2009). However, the incidence rates of the BC are also rapidly increasing in a number of low- and middle-income countries (LMIC) (Forouzanfar et al, 2011), with more than half of all deaths caused by BC globally occurring in these countries (Curado et al (Eds.), 2009; Forouzanfar et al, 2011; International Agency for Research in Cancer, 2008). In LMIC countries, a sizeable proportion of women killed by BC were aged 15-49 years (Forouzanfar et al, 2011).

In the period from the year 1954 to the year 2006 a number of demographic changes took place in Slovenia (population two million) that may have contributed to the increase in the incidence rate of BC in recent decades. Major changes were observed in the size and age of population, in the number of live births annually, in the number of live births per 1,000 population, in total fertility rate, the age of mother at first birth and the age of mother at birth in total. In detail, the population of Slovenia grew from 1,521,485 to 2,008,516 in the period from 1954 to 2006, but simultaneously a decrease was observed in the number of live births annually, in the number of live births per 1,000 population and in total fertility rate (Ilić et al., 2008). On the other hand, an increase was observed in the age of mother at first birth and the age of mother at birth in total in the same period (Ilić et al., 2008). The data about population by sex are available only for the period from mid-1969 on and of all the people living in Slovenia on June 30th of that year, 826,145 were men and 887,877 were women. In mid-2006, 986,876 were men and 1,022,644 were women, and the population of both sexes had been growing older in the decades prior to 2006. A substantial increase in the mean age of women at death was observed in the period from 1961 to 2006, reflecting an overall increase in age in Slovenian population in recent decades (Ilić et al., 2008).

In this report, the authors assess the possible impact of changes in some of the demographic indicators in Slovenia on the increase in the incidence rate of BC and therefore also on the possible role of midwives in the early detection and prevention of BC in the future. With regard to the recent increases of the incidence rates of BC in a number of LMIC countries, it may be plausible to consider the evolution and broadening of the role of midwives in the early detection and prevention of BC in these countries as well.

2. Changes in some of the demographic indicators and simultaneous increase in the incidence rate of breast cancer in recent decades in Slovenia

The data concerning the changes in some of the demographic indicators and simultaneous increase in the incidence rate of BC in Slovenia were collected and downloaded from open access electronic databases of the National Institute of Public Health of the Republic of Slovenia (National Institute of Public Health of the Republic of Slovenia, 2011), Statistical Office of the Republic of Slovenia (Statistical Office of the Republic of Slovenia, 2011), Slora-Slovenia and Cancer (Slora, 2011) of the Cancer Registry of Republic of Slovenia and from some of the similar sources (Cancer Registry of Republic of Slovenia, 2010; Curado et al (Eds.), 2009; Ilić et al., 2008). In this report the data in the figures refer only to the period from 1961 to 2006 since the data from periods earlier than 1961 are subject to limited availability. The data were processed and presented with the use of Excel 97 for Windows software package.

As already mentioned above, BC is the most common type of cancer and most common cause of death from cancer in Slovenia (Cancer Registry of Republic of Slovenia, 2010; Slora 2011). The incidence rate of BC has been increasing constantly in the last five decades (Figure 1). In a large part of this period, from 1961 to 2006, a simultaneous decrease had been observed in the number of live births annually, in the number of live births per 1,000 population and in total fertility rate (Ilić et al, 2008; Slora, 2011; Statistical Office of the Republic of Slovenia, 2011). The number of live births decreased from 31,828 to 18,932 in the period from 1961 to 2006 (Figure 2), the number of live births per 1,000 population decreased from 18.1 to 9.4 (Figure 3), and total fertility rate decreased from 2.26 to 1.31 in the same period (Figure 4). Conversely, for at least a part of this period, from late-seventies and early-eighties onward, the age of mother at first birth and the age of mother at birth in total both increased (Figure 5) (Ilić et al., 2008; Slora, 2011; Statistical Office of the Republic of Slovenia, 2011). The age of mother at first birth increased from 24.7 years in 1961 to 28 years in 2006, the lowest age of mother at first birth in this period was 22.7 years, observed in 1976, and the age of mother at birth in total increased from 27.7 years in 1961 to 29.7 years in 2006, the lowest age of mother at birth in total in this period was 25.3 years, observed in 1979, 1980 and in 1984 (Figure 5). (Ilić et al., 2008; Statistical Office of the Republic of Slovenia, 2011). Finally, the mean age at death of women increased from 59.8 years in 1954 to 78.1 years in 2006 (Figure 6) (Ilić et al., 2008; Slora, 2011; Statistical Office of the Republic of Slovenia, 2011).

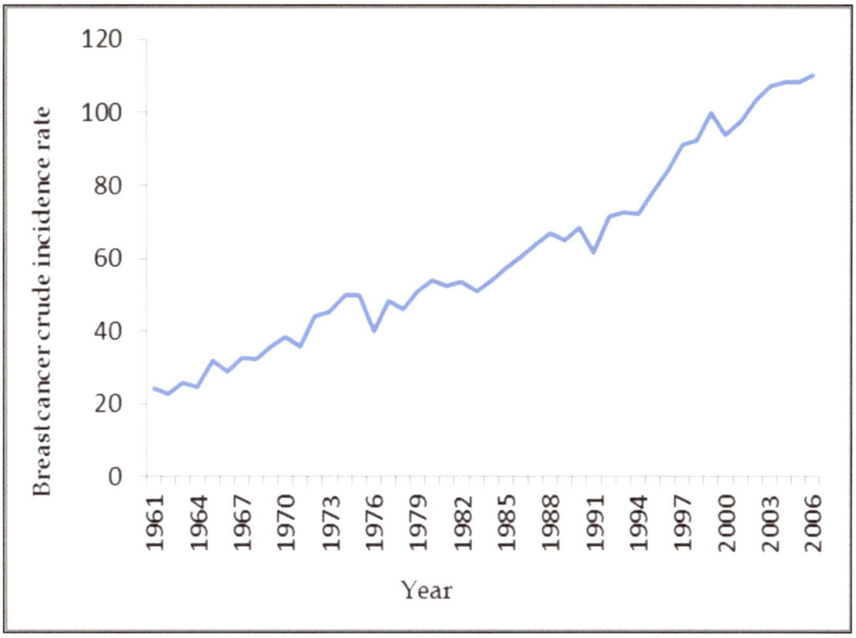

Fig. 1. Breast cancer crude incidence rate (blue line; definition: crude incidence rate is the number of new cases of disease or the number of deceased from the disease, calculated per 100,000 of population-persons, living in observed population in the middle of the time interval, usually one year (Slora, 2011; Statistical Office of the Republic of Slovenia, 2011)) in the period from 1961 to 2006 in Slovenia

Considering the changes in some of the aforementioned demographic factors and the corresponding increase in the incidence rate of BC in Slovenia, it is easy to imagine that these changes represent an increase in the risk of BC in women in the period from 1961 to 2006 in this country. Some additional data about changes in population in Slovenia in the recent decades in the following text may corroborate this notion.

As already suggested, the population of both sexes had aged quite rapidly in Slovenia. In 2006 the mean age of the population overall was 40.7 years; 39 years of men and 42.3 years of women. In the period between 1986 and 2006, the population of Slovenia has on average grown older by 5.6 years, by the end of this period men were on average older by 5.7 years and women by 5.6 years. The mean age of men grew the most between 1997 and 1998, and of women between 2001 and 2002 (Ilić et al., 2008). In 2006 the proportion of young population aged 0-14 years was 14% and the proportion of population aged 65 years or more was 15.7%. In the twenty years from 1986 to 2006 the number of individuals in population aged 0-14 years decreased by more than a third (34.8%) and the number of individuals in population aged 65 years or more increased by more than a half (59%) (Ilić et al, 2008). In just ten years, in the period from 1996 to 2006, the number of women in reproductive age (15-49 years) in Slovenia decreased from 518,335 in 1996 to 476,853 in 2006 (Ilić et al, 2008). In 1954 slightly over a third of children were first-born and almost 20% of mothers had at least four children, while in the last three decades of the period from 1954 to 2006 approximately half of all births were first order births (49.6% in 2006), more than one third of births were second order births (35.8% in 2006), slightly more than 10% were third order births (10.9% in 2006) and only about 3% of births were fourth order births or higher (3.7% in 2006) (Ilić et al., 2008).

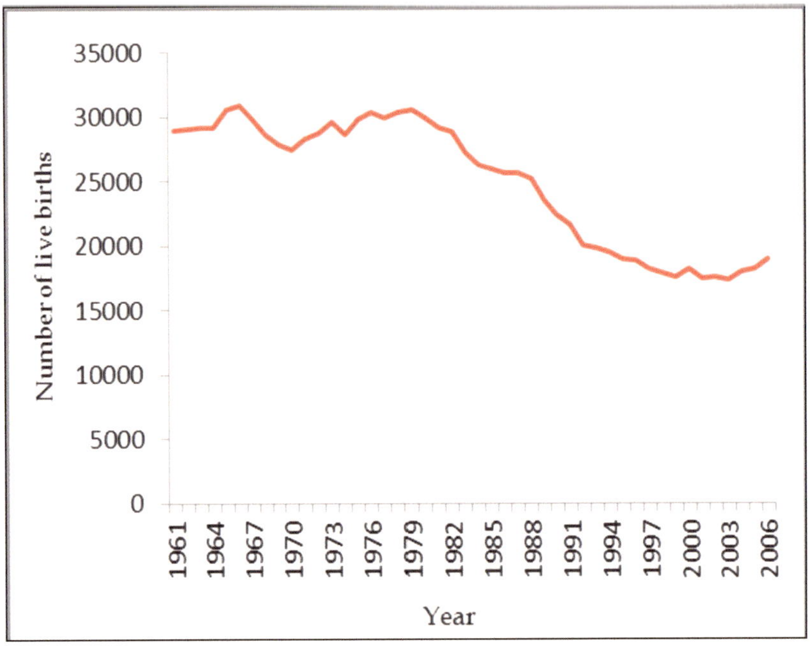

Fig. 2. Number of live births (red line; definition: number of live born children in the calendar year) in the period from 1961 to 2006 in Slovenia

In addition, it was also possible to retrieve some further data, for the period from 1954 to 1961, for the age of mother at first birth and the age of mother at birth in total, both risk factors for BC. Altogether, the age of mother at first birth rose from 24.8 years in the year 1954 to 28.0 years in the year 2006. The age of mother at birth in total rose from 28.4 years in 1954 to 29.7 years in 2006 (Ilić et al, 2008). Postponement of birth of the first child is typical for women of many European Union countries, especially in the lowest-low fertility countries. In some of these countries the trends in postponing of births is so intense that annual increase in the mean age is 0.2 years, with extremely fast postponement occurring in Slovenia, Hungary and the Czech Republic. In the United Kingdom, the mean age of women that gave birth to their children for the first time reached 30 years in 2006 (Ilić et al, 2008).

On the whole, increased risk of BC is associated with female gender, advancing age and age during menstrual life, hormonal factors (early menarche and late menopause), nulliparity and age of over 30 years at first birth, obesity and estrogen therapy after the menopause, harmful drinking of alcohol and history of benign proliferative lesions in the breast (Armstrong & Nguyen, 1999; Bryant, 2004; Cancer Registry of Republic of Slovenia, 2010; Curado et al (Eds.), 2009; Henderson et al, 1996; International Agency for Research in Cancer, 2008; Soerjomataram et al, 2008). Risk of BC is also increased in women with one or more first-degree relatives with BC (Henderson et al, 1996), and with inherited mutations of any one of major genes, like BRCA1, BRCA2 and several others (Armstrong & Nguyen, 1999; International Agency for Research in Cancer, 2008).

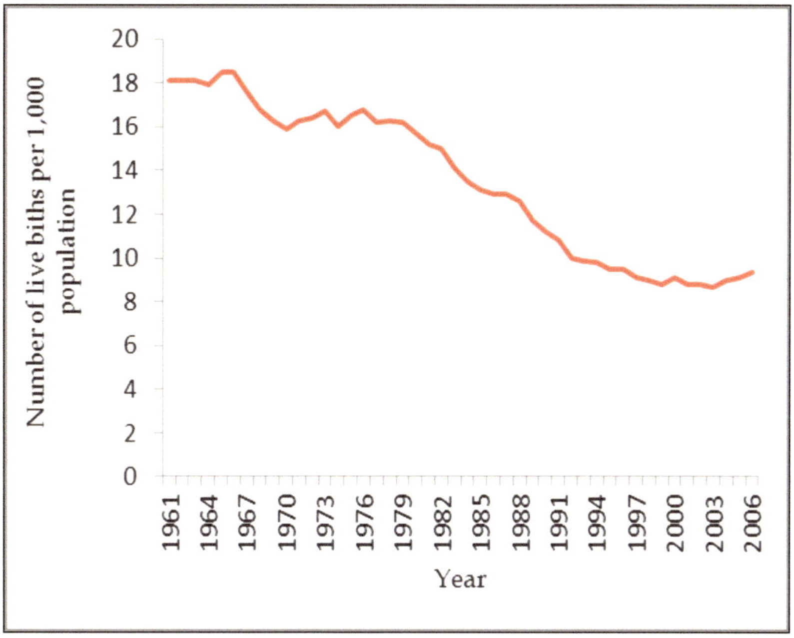

Fig. 3. Number of live births per 1,000 population (red line; definition: ratio between the number of live born children in the calendar year and the same mid-year population, multiplied by 1,000 (Ilić et al., 2008)) in the period from 1961 to 2006 in Slovenia

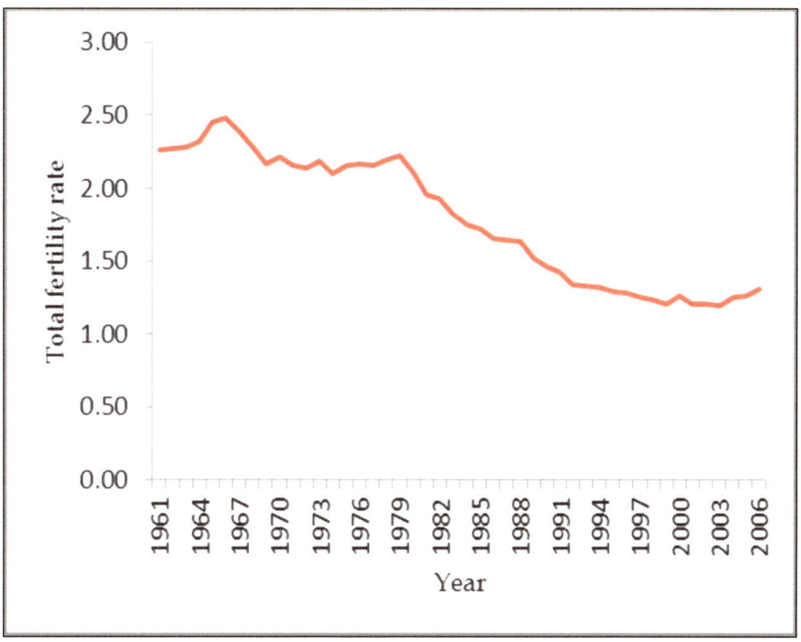

Fig. 4. Total fertility rate (red line; definition: the average number of live born children per one woman in reproductive age (15-49 years) in the calendar year (Ilić et al., 2008)) in the period from 1961 to 2006 in Slovenia

It may be of particular interest that the number of women diagnosed with BC in the year 2008 in Slovenia is slightly lower than in the year 2007, when the incidence rate of BC reached 112.9 cases per 100,000 and when BC was diagnosed in 1,156 women (Cancer Registry of Republic of Slovenia, 2010; Slora, 2011). However, the incidence rates of BC are still notably lower in Slovenia than in the United States of America and in a number of other developed European Union countries. It remains to be seen if this small decrease in the incidence rate of BC in Slovenia represents the same type of trend as observed in the United States of America, where the incidence rates of BC decreased by approximately two percent annually in the period from 1999 to 2005 (Centers for Disease Control and Prevention, 2007; Kerlikowske et al, 2007). Later analysis showed that the incidence rate for BC stabilized in the period from 2003 to 2007, following a sharp decrease between 2002 and 2003 observed in women aged 50 years or more (DeSantis et al, 2011a, 2011b), that was associated with the decrease in the use of postmenopausal hormonal replacement therapy (DeSantis et al, 2011b; Kohler et al. 2011; Ravdin et al, 2007).

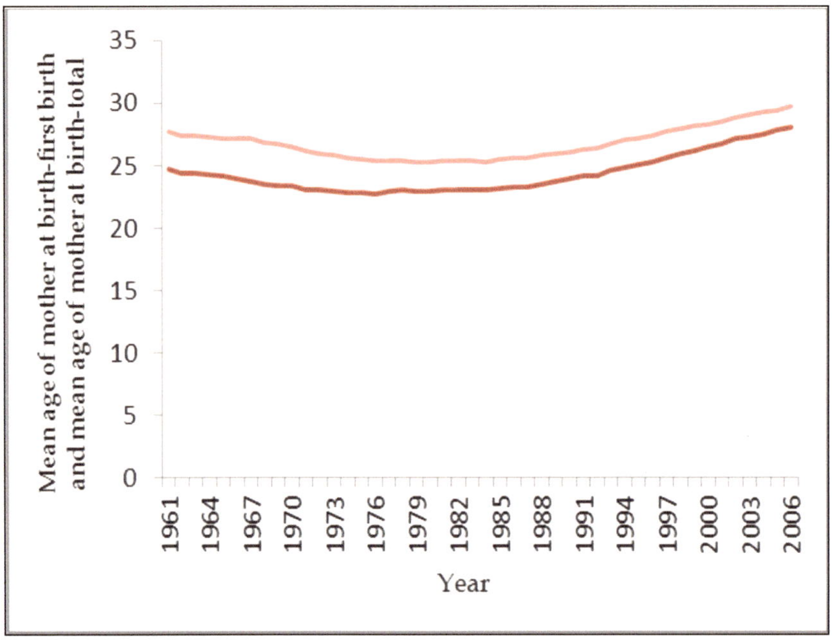

Fig. 5. Mean age mother at first birth (dark red line) and mean age of mother at birth-total (light red line) in the period from 1961 to 2006 in Slovenia

All these data to point to changes in the quantity and quality of the work performed at present by midwives employed in the thirteen maternity wards and maternity hospitals, and elsewhere in Slovenia (National Institute of Public Health of the Republic of Slovenia, 2011). The possible role of midwives in the early detection and prevention of BC in the future should thus be carefully appraised and evaluated.

3. Midwives and breast cancer screening

Study of midwifery has a long and distinguished tradition in Slovenia. The first School for midwives was established in 1753 in Ljubljana, the capital of Slovenia, following the decree issued by Maria Theresa, Empress of Austria, sovereign of all Slovenian lands at that time. Similar Schools for midwives were later also established in Graz, Celovec (Klagenfurt) and Trst (Trieste), all of them at least partly serving the Slovenian-speaking population. After 1924 Midwifery school in Ljubljana remained the only institution which educated midwives in Slovenia. At present the first-cycle degree Professional Higher Education Study Programme Midwifery at the Faculty of Health Sciences at the University of Ljubljana lasts three years (six semesters) and 30 students enrol in the programme each year. The majority of the enrolled students finish the study program and complete their study with a diploma work (Skoberne et al, 2011; Stanek Zidarič et al., 2009).

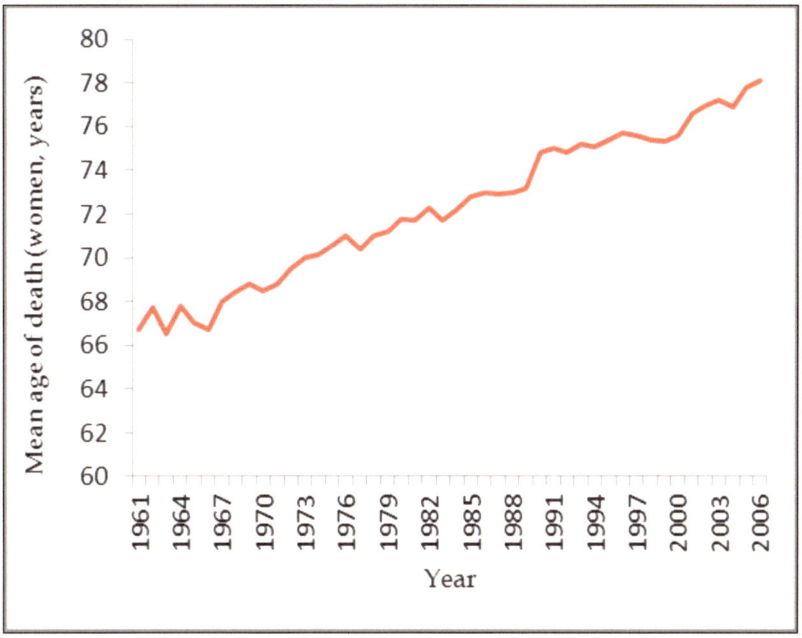

Fig. 6. Mean age of death in women (red line) in the period from 1961 to 2006 in Slovenia

Although it is not particularly emphasized in their curriculum (Stanek Zidarič et al., 2009; World Health Organization & WHO Regional Office for Europe, 2001), midwifery students at the Faculty of Health Sciences in Ljubljana get a reasonable amount of insight into anatomy, histology and physiology of breasts, as well as into incidence, clinical and pathological characteristics, treatment and mortality of BC. They also learn some of the fundamentals about how to perform breast self-examination (BSE) and clinical breast examination (CBE) (Plesničar et al., 2004a; Plesničar et al., 2010; Stanek Zidarič et al., 2009). As a result, midwifery students have a favourable attitude toward BSE, they are of opinion that teaching BSE helps in detection of BC, and that teaching other women how to practice BSE ought to be one of their duties. They are also optimistic in their views of development and efficacy of BC detection and treatment in the future. This sort of attitude toward BC and BSE may have emerged from their specific education and from their inherent motivation to learn as much as possible about clinical, psychological and other problems that affect women with this disease (Plesničar et al., 2004a; Plesničar et al., 2010). All these qualities make them better informed about BC than other women (Budden, 1999; Fischer et al, 2003;

Frank et al, 2000; Gigerenzer et al, 2009; Jirojwong & MacLennan, 2002; Plesničar et al., 2004a; Plesničar et al., 2010). It should also be taken into account that due to their specific education and positive attitude toward BSE, midwifery students should be at the end of their study able to teach BSE to other women and perform CBE quite efficiently (Boulos et al, 2005; Miller et al., 2000; Mittra et al, 2010; Plesničar et al., 2004a; Plesničar et al., 2010).

In the majority of developed countries, including Slovenia, the emphasis is on the use of mammography screening tests focused on early BC detection. These tests enable the discovery of the disease in the early stages of its clinical development, thus improving the chances of longer survival of BC patients (Armstrong & Nguyen, 1999; Dora-državni presejalni program za raka dojk, 2011; Frank et al, 2009; U.S. Preventive Services Task Force. 2009). In a number of studies, however, mammography screening has been shown to reduce breast cancer mortality significantly only for women aged 50–74 years. No benefit has been shown for CBE or BSE (Gøtzsche & Nielsen, 2011; Jekel et al, 1996; Nelson et al, 2009). In addition, some of the studies have, among other problems, also pointed to disagreements about mammography screening tests' efficacy (Gøtzsche & Nielsen, 2011). Harms of BC mammography screening were found to include false-positive results, biopsies and repeated imaging in women without cancer, risks of unnecessary treatment, increased radiation exposure and psychological damage (Gøtzsche & Nielsen, 2011; Meissner et al, 2011; U.S. Preventive Services Task Force, 2009; Welch & Black, 2010). Contrariwise, in Canadian National Breast Screening Study-2 trial mammography with CBE was compared to CBE alone in women aged 50-59 years and no difference in mortality from BC was observed between the two approaches at 13 years (Miller et al, 2000). These controversies have led to suggestions that decisions about participation in mammography screening tests for women should be made on an individualized basis (Berlin & Hall, 2010; Hall, 2009; Meissner et al, 2011; Peres, 2010; Plesničar et al, 2010). The approach that requires work with women on an individual basis should certainly include greater sharing of information and decision making between patient or client and health expert, be that midwife, physician or nurse (Berlin & Hall, 2010; Hall, 2009; Peres, 2010).

In Slovenia primary health care includes specialists in family medicine, paediatrics, psychiatry and gynaecology (Ministry of Health & Government of Republic of Slovenia, 2011b; National Institute of Public Health of the Republic of Slovenia, 2011; Statistical Office of the Republic of Slovenia, 2011). In the year 2011 a number of family practices were upgraded to referral practices, in effect multidisciplinary teams, each one comprising a specialist in family medicine, a nurse and a certified nurse that perform certain activities in accordance with her/his jurisdiction and responsibilities. The aim of such referral practices is to increase quality, safety and cost effectiveness in patient treatment by transferring a number of tasks to the primary level. It is anticipated that each referral practice is involved in optimal integrated care adhering to chronic patient treatment protocols, prevention and optimal use of laboratory services of at least four of the following chronic conditions and treatments: heart failure, chronic obstructive pulmonary disease, asthma, depression, diabetes, benign hypertrophy of the prostate, thyroid diseases and anti-coagulation treatment (Ministry of Health & Government of Republic of Slovenia, 2011b).

Following the aforementioned model of referral practices, it could probably be relatively easy to establish multidisciplinary teams that would among other activities also focus on early detection and prevention of BC. Each such team could comprise a specialist in gynaecology and obstetrics, a midwife and/or a nurse. In some circumstances, for example those distinctive of LMIC countries, midwives could perform their specific activities associated with BC alone. At least in the beginning, midwives could perform CBE as recommended in prevailing guidelines (Boulos et al, 2005; Meissner et al, 2011; Mittra et al, 2010; Plesničar et al, 2010; U.S. Preventive Services Task Force, 2009). Besides performing CBE with or without mammography, the activity of midwives could expand to informing women about breast health awareness (BHA). For women, accepting BHA would mean getting unbiased information about a wide range of breast problems such as breast pain and tenderness, breast asymmetry, nipple discharge, breasts considered to be too small or too large, or about breast lumps, bumps and thickenings (Mitchell, 2002). It would also mean being able to recognize normal appearance and structure of breasts during different periods of menstrual cycle and with regard to pregnancy and age, to recognize undue changes and inform midwife and physician in the multidisciplinary team about them immediately so they could refer these women to mammography tests when necessary (Mitchell, 2002; Plesničar et al., 2004b). Although BSE does not decrease BC mortality (Semiglazov et al, 2004; Thomas et al, 2002; U.S. Preventive Services Task Force, 2009), it can be regarded as an essential component of BHA that may contribute to early BC detection (Mitchell, 2002; Plesničar et al., 2010). Breast self-examination is not much different from what the concept of BHA includes (Dowle et al, 1987; Philip et al, 1984; Plesničar et al., 2010) and in some opinions BHA should broaden the role of BSE (Austoker, 2003; Plesničar et al., 2010). The easiest way to increase BHA could thus be to teach BSE, and in this manner the role of midwives in early BC detection would be given even more prominence (Miller et al., 2000; Plesničar et al., 2004a, Plesničar et al., 2010).

Further on, midwives could take part in BC risk factor reduction or elimination and some other specific health promotion activities, all of them part of primary prevention, that would focus on introducing subtle and hardly measurable changes in women's and population's way of living with the aim of decreasing BC incidence in the longer term in Slovenia and elsewhere. These activities could include education about health behaviour modification with prolonged lactation, healthy lifestyle with regular physical activity, and proper nutrition to prevent obesity and harmful consumption of alcohol. For postmenopausal women these activities could also include the information about the risks of the use of hormonal replacement therapy (Armstrong & Nguyen, 1999; Anderson et al 2008, DeSantis et al, 2011b; Henderson et al, 1996; Jekel et al, 1996; Kohler et al. 2011; Ravdin et al, 2007). All these activities and procedures would be carried out on an individual basis, in time gradually replacing mammography screening with individual BC case finding (Jekel et al, 1996).

Finally, it may be appropriate to cite comments of Otis Brawley, MD, chief medical officer of the American Cancer Society, with regard to prostate cancer screening and simply substitute the word breast for prostate (Berlin & Hall, 2010) and make a mention of midwives in the context: adequately trained and experienced midwives could help every woman take an informed decision about what is right for her personally after hearing a balanced presentation of potential benefits and risks of screening. All in the medical and advocacy communities should respect that choice (Brawley, 2009, as cited in Berlin & Hall, 2010)

4. Discussion

The changes in demographics and in the incidence rate of BC in the last decades surely represent serious and important challenges for health care system in Slovenia. Despite the content and context of these changes in Slovenia, the number of midwifery graduates, the contents of midwifery students' curriculum, the numbers of maternity wards and maternity hospitals have remained more or less constant and without sensible changes in recent years.

All the data about changes in demographic indicators with potential impact on the increase of BC incidence rates in Slovenia may not have been shown in this report. However, the changes in number of live births, number of live births per 1,000 population, total fertility rate, age of mother at first birth and age of mother at birth in total, and mean age of death in women in the period from 1961 to 2006, certainly suggest that there are now many more women exposed to the risk of BC than four or five decades ago (Armstrong & Nguyen, 1999; Bryant, 2004; Curado et al (Eds.), 2009; Henderson et al, 1996; International Agency for Research in Cancer, 2008; Soerjomataram et al 2008). The changes in demographic indicators and the increase in the incidence rate of BC in Slovenia in the last decades should at the very least stimulate a debate about changes in priorities in activities of midwives and related experts and specialists today and in the future. One of the future priorities for midwives could be early detection and prevention of BC that would include informing women about BHA and about risk factors of BC on an individual basis. In Slovenia and some other countries midwives already occupy a central position in education of young women about sexual and reproductive health, family planning and contraception (Ministry of Health & Government of Republic of Slovenia, 2011a). It should not be difficult to imagine the midwives establishing a trustful and confidential professional relationship with women in late teens or early twenties, informing them about BHA, BSE, CBE, BC, age adjusted BC risk factors and their reduction or elimination, performing CBE according to guidelines and later in their lives informing them about BC mammography screening programs.

About two thirds of all cancer cases are diagnosed in economically developed countries and about one third in LMIC countries (Forouzanfar et al, 2011; International Agency for Research in Cancer, 2008; Mellstedt, 2006). In the year 2010 the majority of women with BC in economically and industrially developed countries were aged 50 years or more. However, in developing countries there were twice as many women with BC aged 15-49 years than in developed countries, with the incidence rate of BC overall rising rapidly (Forouzanfar et al, 2011; International Agency for Research in Cancer, 2008; Mittra, 2011; Yeole & Kurkure, 2003). In view of these developments, it is agreed that mammography is not an appropriate BC screening test for LMIC countries. It is expensive, technologically complex and requires highly skilled experts and quality control (Berlin & Hall, 2010; Frank et al, 2000; Harford, 2011; Mittra, 2011; Nelson et al, 2009; U.S. Preventive Services Task Force, 2009). Conversely, CBE is relatively easy and inexpensive to perform (Mittra, 2011; Nelson et al, 2009). However, its effectiveness in reducing BC mortality is still regarded as controversial (Nelson et al, 2009), although the results of Canadian National Breast Screening Study-2 strongly suggest such an effect (Miller et al, 2000; Mittra, 2011). Two major randomized trials in Mumbai and Cairo comparing CBE and no screening are now addressing this dilemma. In Mumbai CBE and education are performed by female health workers who underwent five months of additional training, while in Cairo examinations are performed by female physicians who received two months of special training (Boulos et al, 2005; Mittra et al, 2010). In both studies there have been difficulties in assuring follow-up, a problem in many cases due to low levels of health awareness and motivation in screened communities (Miller, 2008; Mittra et al, 2010; Mittra, 2011). It is intriguing to speculate that this problem may otherwise not be encountered in Slovenia or other developed countries. These two studies may confirm the effectiveness of CBE and its use in LMIC countries may obviate the perceived need for establishing complex mammography screening programs, especially since a large proportion of women diagnosed with BC in these countries are aged 15-49 years.

The results of Mumbai and Cairo studies may strengthen the arguments for use of CBE by midwives in Slovenia and elsewhere. Altogether, the activities of midwives working with women on an individual basis, whether alone or as a part of a multidisciplinary team in a referral practice, including informing and teaching women about BHA, giving other information and performing CBE, could be described as lifetime breast health monitoring, a development of practice described already more than thirty years ago (Breslow & Somers, 1977).

5. Conclusion

It is imperative to understand the need to change and supplement secondary prevention of BC from mammography screening to individual BC case finding that would include mammography when necessary. In the future, individual BC case finding should be further developed to lifetime breast health monitoring, making midwives role in multidisciplinary teams indispensable. In certain surroundings and circumstances, especially in LMIC countries, midwives could also operate alone. In Slovenia and other parts of the world, including LMIC countries, where increasing incidence rate of BC and demographic changes represent a serious public health issue, their skills, proficiency, positive attitudes and goodwill should not be left unused.

6. References

Armstrong, B.K. & Nguyen, H.L. (1999). Breast cancer, In: *Cancer Facts. A Concise Oncology Text*, Bishop, J.F., Editor, pp. 127-132, Interwood Academic Publishers, ISBN 90-5702-470-5, Amsterdam, The Netherlands

Anderson, B.O.; Yip, C.H.; Smith, R.A.; Shyyan, R.; Sener, S.F.; Eniu, A.; Carlson, R.W.; Azavedo, R. & Harford, J. Guideline implementation for breast healthcare in low-income and middle-income countries. Overview of the Breast Health Initiative Global Summit 2007. *Cancer*, Vol. 113, No. 8, (June 2008), pp. 2221-2243, ISSN 1097-0142

Austoker, J. (2003). Breast self examination. *British Medical Journal*, Vol. 326, No. 7379, (January 2003), pp. 1-2, ISSN 1468-5833

Berlin, L. & Hall, F.M. (2010). More mammography muddle: emotions, politics, science, costs, and polarization. *Radiology*, Vol. 255, No. 2, (May 2010), pp. 311-316, ISSN 1527-1315

Boulos, S.; Gadallah, M.; Neguib, S.; Essam, E.; Youssef, A.; Costa, A.; Mittra, I. & Miller, A.B. (2005). Breast screening in the emerging world: high prevalence of breast cancer in Cairo. *Breast (Edinburgh, Scotland)*, Vol. 14, No. 5, (October 2005), pp. 340-346, ISSN 0960-9776

Bryant, H. (2004). Breast cancer in Canadian women. *BMC Women's Health*, Vol. 4, Suppl. 1, (August 2004), pp. S12, ISSN 1472-6874

Budden, L. (1999). Student nurses' breast self-examination health beliefs, attitudes, knowledge, and performance during the first year of a preregistration degree program. *Cancer Nursing*, Vol. 22, No. 6, (December 1999), pp. 430-437, ISSN 1538-9804

Cancer Registry of Republic of Slovenia. (2010). *Cancer Incidence in Slovenia; 2007. Report No. 49*, Institute of Oncology, ISSN 1318-2471, Ljubljana, Slovenia

Centers for Disease Control and Prevention. (2007). Decline in breast cancer incidence-United States, 1999-2003. *MMWR. Morbidity and Mortality Weekly Report*, Vol. 56, No. 22, (June 2007). pp. 549-553, ISSN 0149-2195

Curado, M.P.; Edwards, B.; Shin, H.R.; Storm, H.; Ferlay, J.; Heanue, M. & Boyle, P. (Eds.). *Cancer Incidence in Five Continents. Volume IX. IARC Scientific Publications No. 160.* International Agency for Research on Cancer, ISBN 978-92-832-2160, Lyon, France

DeSantis, C.; Howlader, N.; Cronin, K.A. & Jemal, A. (2011) Breast cancer incidence rates in US women are no longer declining. *Cancer epidemiology, Biomarkers & Prevention : A Publication of the American Association for Cancer Research, Cosponsored by the American Society of Preventive Oncology*, Vol. 20, No. 5, (May 2011), pp. 733-739, ISSN 1055-9965

DeSantis, C.; Siegel, R.; Bandi, P. & Jemal, A. (2011). Breast cancer statistics, 2011. *CA: A Cancer Journal for Clinicians*, Vol. 61, No. 6, (November/December, 2011), pp. 408-418, ISSN 1542-4863

Dora-državni presejalni program za raka dojk. (2011). Presejanje za raka dojk. In: Dora-državni presejalni program za raka dojk, Date of access: October 25th, 2011, Available from: <http://dora.onko-i.si/presejanje_za_raka_dojk/index.html>

Dowle, C.S.; Mitchell, A.; Elston, C.W.; Roebuck, E.J.; Hinton, C.P.; Holliday, H. & Blamey, R.W. (1987). Preliminary results of the Nottingham breast self-examination education programme. *The British Journal of Surgery*, Vol. 74, No. 3, (March 1987), pp. 217-219, ISSN 1365-2168

Fischer, V.; Pabst, R. & Nave, H. (2003). Seminar in breast self-examination for female medical students integrated into a human gross anatomy course. *Clinical Anatomy (New York, N.Y.)*, Vol. 16, No. 2, (March 2003), pp.160-164, ISSN 0897-3806

Forouzanfar, M.H.; Foreman, K.J.; Delossantos, A.M.; Lozano, R.; Lopez, A.D.; Murray, C.J.L. & Naghavi, M. (2011). Breast and cervical cancer in 187 countries between 1980 and 2010: a systematic analysis. *The Lancet*, Vol. 378, No. 9801, (October 2011), pp. 1461-1484, ISSN 0099-5355

Frank, E.; Rimer, B.K.; Brogan, D. & Elon, L. (2000). U.S. women physicians' personal and clinical breast cancer screening practices. *Journal of Women's Health & Gender Based Medicine*, Vol. 9, No. 7, (September 2000), pp. 791-801, ISSN 1524-6094

Gigerenzer, G.; Mata, J. & Frank, R. (2009). Public knowledge of benefits of breast and prostate cancer screening in Europe. *Journal of National Cancer Institute*, Vol. 101, No. 8, (April 2009), pp. 1216-1220, ISSN 1460-2105

Gøtzsche, P.C. & Nielsen, M. (2011). Screening for breast cancer with mammography (review). *Cochrane Database of Systematic Reviews*, No. 1, (January 2011), pp. 1-47, ISSN 1469-493X

Hall, F.M. (2009). The radiology report of the future. *Radiology*, Vol. 251, No. 2, (May 2009), pp. 313-316, ISSN 1527-1315

Harford, J.B. (2011). Breast cancer early detection in low-income and middle-income countries: do what you can versus one size fits all. *The Lancet Oncology*, Vol. 12, No. 3, (March 2011), pp. 306-312, ISSN 1470-2045

Henderson, B.E.; Pike, M.C.; Bernstein, L. & Ross, R.K. (1996). *Breast Cancer*, In: Cancer Epidemiology and Prevention, Schottenfeld, D. & Fraumeni, J.F., Editors, pp. 1022-1039, Oxford University Press, New York, New York, USA

Ilić, M.; Kalin, K.; Povhe, J.; Šter, D. & Žnidaršič, T. (2008). *Population of Slovenia 2006. Results of Surveys No. 831/2008.* Statistical Office of the Republic of Slovenia, ISBN 978-961-239-170-9, Ljubljana, Slovenia

International Agency for Research in Cancer. (2008). Breast Cancer Incidence and Mortality Worldwide in 2008. Summary, In: *Globocan 2008. Cancer Incidence and Mortality Worldwide in 2008,* Date of access November 8th, 2011, Available from: <http://globocan.iarc.fr/factsheets/cancers/breast.asp>

Jekel, J.F.; Elmore, J.G. & Katz, D.L. (1996). *Epidemiology, Statistics and Preventive Medicine, 1st edition.* WB Saunders Company, ISBN 0-7216-5258-1, Philadelphia, Pennsylvania, USA

Jirojwong, S. & MacLennan R. (2003). Health beliefs, perceived self-efficacy, and breast self-examination among Thai migrants in Brisbane. *Journal of Advanced Nursing,* Vol. 41, No. 3, (February 2003), pp. 241-249, ISSN 1365-2648

Kerlikowske, K.; Miglioretti, D.L.; Buist, D.S.; Walker, R.; Carney, P.A. & National Cancer Institute-Sponsored Breast Cancer Surveillance Consortium. (2007). Declines in invasive breast cancer and use of postmenopausal hormone therapy in a screening mammography population. *Journal of National Cancer Institute*, Vol. 99, No. 7, (September 2007), pp.1335-1339, ISSN 1460-2105

Kohler, B.A.; Ward, E.; McCarthy, B.J.; Schymura, M.J.; Ries, L.A.G.; Eheman, C.; Jemal, A.; Anderson, R.M.; Ajani, U.A. & Edwards, B.K. (2011). Annual report to the nation on the status of cancer, 1975-2007, featuring tumors of the brain and other nervous system. *Journal of National Cancer Institute*, Vol. 103, No. 9, (May 2011), pp. 1-23, ISSN 1460-2105

Meissner, H.I.; Klabunde, C.N.; Han, P.K.; Benard, V.B. & Breen, N. (2011). Breast cancer screening beliefs, recommendations, and practices. Primary Care physicians in the United States. *Cancer,* Vol. 117, No. 14. (July 2011), pp. 3101-3111, ISSN 1097-0142

Mellstedt, H. (2006). Cancer initiatives in developing countries. *Annals of Oncology*, Vol. 17, Suppl. 8, (June 2006). pp. viii24-viii31, ISSN 1569-8041

Miller, A.B.; To, T.; Baines, C.J. & Wall, C. (2000). Canadian National Breast Screening Study-2: 13-year results of a randomized trial in women aged 50-59 years. *Journal of National Cancer Institute*, Vol. 92, No. 18, (September 2000), pp. 1490-1499, ISSN 1460-2105

Miller, A.B. (2008). Practical applications for clinical breast examination (CBE) and breast self-examination (BSE) in screening and early detection of breast cancer. *Breast Care (Basel, Switzerland)*, Vol. 3, No. 1, (February 2008), pp. 17-20, ISSN 1661-3791

Ministry of Health & Government of Republic of Slovenia. (2011a). Date of Access: October 26th, 2011, Available from: <http://www.mz.gov.si/si>

Ministry of Health & Government of Republic of Slovenia. (2011b). Referenčna ambulanta. In: *publikacije in druga gradiva*, Date of Access: October 23rd, 2011, Available from: <http://www.mz.gov.si/si/mz_za_vas/zdravstveno_varstvo/referencne_ambulante/

Mitchell, A. (2002). Breast health awareness, In: *Evidence-based health promotion*. 4th edition, E.R. Perkins, I. Simnet, L. Wright, Editors, pp. 266-274, John Wiley & Sons, ISBN 0-471-97851-5, Chichester, England

Mittra, I.; Mishra, G.A.; Singh, S.; Aranke, S.; Notani, P.; Badwe, R.; Miller, A.B.; Daniel, E.E.; Gupta, S.; Uplap, P.; Thakur, M.H.; Ramani, S.; Kerkar, R.; Ganesh, B. & Shastri, S.S. (2010). A cluster randomized, controlled trial of breast and cervix cancer screening in Mumbai, India: methodology and interim results after three rounds of screening. *International Journal of Cancer. Journal International du Cancer*, Vol. 126, No. 4, (February 2010), pp. 976-984, 0020-7136

Mittra, I. (2011). Breast cancer screening in developing countries. *Preventive Medicine*, Vol. 53, No. 3, (June 2011), pp. 121-122, ISSN 1096-0260

National Institute of Public Health of the Republic of Slovenia. (2011). In: *Podatkovne zbirke-zdravstveni statistični podatki*, Date of access October 21st, 2011, Available from: <http://www.ivz.si/Mp.aspx?ni=46&pi=5&_5_id=1771&_5_PageIndex=0&_5_groupId=185&_5_newsCategory=&_5_action=ShowNewsFull&pl=46-5.0.>

Nelson, H.D.; Tyne, K.; Naik, A.; Bougatsos, C.; Chan, B.; Nygren, P. & Humphrey, L. (2009). *Screening for breast cancer: systematic evidence review update for the US preventive services task force. Evidence Review Update, No. 74.* AHRQ Publication No. 10-05142-EF-1. Rockville, Maryland, USA

Peres, J. (2010). Mammography screening: after the storm, calls for more personalized approaches. *Journal of National Cancer Institute*, Vol. 102, No. 1, (January 2010), ISSN 1460-2105

Philip, J.; Harris, W.G.; Flaherty, C.; Joslin, C.A.; Rustage, J.H. & Wijesinghe, D.P. (1984). Breast self-examination: clinical results from a population-based prospective study. *British Journal of Cancer*, Vol. 50, No. 1, (July 1984), pp. 7-12, ISSN 0007-0920

Plesničar, A.; Goličnik, M. & Kralj, B. (2004a). Midwifery students and breast self-examination. *The Breast Journal*, Vol. 10, No. 6, (November/December 2004), pp. 560, ISSN 1075-122X

Plesničar, A.; Kovač, V. & Kralj, B. (2004b). Breast cancer and breast health awareness as an evolving health promotion concept. *Radiology and Oncology*, Vol. 38, No. 1, (March 2004), pp. 27-34, ISSN 1318-2099

Plesničar, A.; Goličnik, M.; Kirar Fazarinc, I.; Kralj, B.; Kovač, V. & Kores Plesničar, B. (2010). Attitudes of midwifery students towards teaching breast self-examination. *Radiology and Oncology*, Vol. 44, No. 1, (March 2010), pp. 52-56, ISSN 1318-2099

Ravdin, P.M.; Kronin, K.A.; Howlader, N.; Berg, C.D.; Chlebowski, R.T.; Feuer, E.J.; Edwards, B.K. & Berry, D.A. (2007). The decrease in breast-cancer incidence in 2003 in the United States. *New England Journal of Medicine*, Vol. 356, No. 16, (April 2007), pp. 1670-1674, ISSN 0028-4793

Semiglazov, V.F.; Manikhas, A.G.; Moiseenko, V.M.; Protsenko, S.A.; Kharikova, R.S.; Seleznev, I.K.; Popova, R.T.; Migmanova, N.Sh.; Orlov, A.A.; Barash, N.Iu.; Ivanova, O.A. & Ivanov V.G. (2003). Results of a prospective randomized investigation [Russia (St. Petersburg)/WHO] to evaluate the significance of self-evaluation for the early detection of breast cancer. *Voprosy Onkologii*, Vol. 49, No. 4; (April 2003), pp. 434-441, ISSN 0507-3758

Slora-Slovenia and Cancer. (2011). Slovenian data. In: *Website on cancer information in Slovenia and other countries*, Date of access: October 12th, 2011, Available from: <http://www.slora.si/en/analizaslo>

Skoberne, M.; Mivšek A.P.; Zakšek, T. & Skubic, M. (2011). Midwifery. In: *Faculty of health sciences*. 1st edition, D. Rugelj, Editor, pp. 31-37, Faculty of Health Sciences, ISBN 978-961-6808-22-4, Ljubljana, Slovenia

Soerjomataram, I.; Pukkala, E.; Brenner, H. & Coebergh, J.W. (2008). On the avoidability of breast cancer in industrialized societies: Older mean age at first birth as an indicator of excess breast cancer risk. *Breast Cancer Research and Treatment*, Vol. 111, No. 2, (September 2008), pp. 297-302, ISSN 0167-6806

Stanek Zidarič, T.; Mivšek, A.P.; Skoberne, M.; Skubic, M. & Zakšek, T. (2009). *Professional higher education study programme 1st cycle degree – midwifery*, University of Ljubljana, Faculty of Health Sciences, ISBN 978-961-6063-99-9, Ljubljana, Slovenia

Statistical Office of the Republic of Slovenia. (2011). In: *Demography and social statistics*, Date of access: October 19th, 2011, Available from: <http://www.stat.si/eng/tema_ demografsko.asp?SklopID=3>

Thomas, D.B.; Gao, D.L.; Ray, R.M.; Wang, W.W.; Allison, C.J.; Chen, F.L.; Porter, P.; Hu, Y.W.; Zhao, G.L.; Pan, L.D.; Li, W.; Wu, C.; Coriaty, Z.; Evans, I.; Lin, M.G.; Stalsberg, H. & Self, S.G. (2002).Randomized trial of breast self-examination in Shanghai: final results. *Journal of National Cancer Institute*; Vol. 94, No. 19, (October 2002), pp. 1445-1457, ISSN 1460-2105

U.S. Preventive Services Task Force. (2009). Screening for breast cancer: U.S. preventive services task force recommendation statement. *Annals of Internal Medicine*, Vol. 151; No. 10, (November 2009), pp. 716-726, ISSN 1539-3704

Welch, H.G. & Black, W.C. (2010). Overdiagnosis in cancer. *Journal of National Cancer Institute*, Vol. 102, No. 9, (April 2010), pp. 605-613, ISSN 1460-2105

World Health Organization; WHO Regional Office for Europe. (2001). *Nurses and Midwives for Health. WHO European Strategy for Nursing and Midwifery Education* (1st edition), WHO Regional Office for Europe, ISBN 92-890-1191-2, Copenhagen, Denmark

Yip, C.H.; Cazap, E.; Anderson, B.O.; Bright, K.L.; Caleffi, M.; Cardoso, F.; Elzawawy, A.M.; Harford, J.B.; Krygier, G.D.; Masood, S.; Murillo, R.; Muse, I.M.; Otero, I.V.; Passman, L.J.; Santini, L.A.; Corrêa Ferreira da Silva, R.; Thomas, D.B.; Torres, S.; Zheng, Y. & Khaled, H.M. (2011). Breast cancer management in middle-resource countries (MRCs): Consensus statement from the Breast Health Global Initiative. *Breast (Edinburgh, Scotland)*, Vol. 20, Suppl. 2, (April 2011), pp. S12-S19, ISSN 0960-9776

Yeole, B.B. & Kurkure A. P. (2003). An epidemiological assessment of inceasing incidence and trends in breast cancer in Mumbai and other sites in India, during the last two decades. *Asian Pacific Journal of Cancer Prevention,* Vol. 4, No. 1, (January-March 2003), pp. 51-56, ISSN 1513-7363

6

Chemokines & Their Receptors in Non-Small Cell Lung Cancer Detection

Nadeem Sheikh*, Tasleem Akhtar and Nyla Riaz
Department of Zoology, University of the Punjab, Q-A campus, Lahore, Pakistan

1. Introduction

One of the most commonly diagnosed cancers is non-small cell lung cancer (NSCLC), which is the leading cause of lung cancer related deaths throughout the world [1;2]. NSCLC is an aggressive tumor having poor surveillance. Patients with NSCLC have only 15% or less five year survival rate [3]. Many genetic abnormalities involved in the pathogenesis of NSCLC e.g. mutation in the *p53* gene a tumor suppressor gene.

Chemokines; a superfamily of cytokines, low molecular weight (8-10kDa) proteins, are chemo-attractants for leukocytes and chemokines contains more than 40 ligands and 20 receptors [4;5]. Chemokines can be grouped into four sub families on the basis of the first two of four conserved cysteine residues, functional activity and receptor binding properties and are abbreviated as C, CC, CXC and CX3C.

C chemokines or γ chemokines contains only two cysteines residues; one cysteine present at amino terminal and second present downstream, present in thymus and are chemoattractant for T cell precursors.

CC chemokines are also called as ß-chemokines, have two adjacent cysteines at their N-terminal. These proteins induce the migration of immune cells, mainly dendritic cells, natural killer cells and monocytes.

CXC chemokines or α-chemokines are those in which single amino acid separates two adjacent cysteines present at N- terminal, thus have an "X" in their name. These are divided into two groups, ELR positive and ELR-negative.

In CX3C chemokines or d-chemokines, two cysteines are separated by three amino acids. It acts in an autocrine manner i.e. secreted and act on the same cell.

Chemokines have an important role in pro-inflammatory as well as non-inflammatory cell homing [6]. Chemokines cause the migration of leukocytes to inflammatory sites and also play role in the hematopoietic stem cells regulation, angiogenesis and the extracellular matrix. This super-family also plays additional role in diverse fields including development, immunology and cancer.

---

* Corresponding Author

Chemokines also play an important role in the neoplastic transformation of a cell, encourage angiogenesis, tumor colonial expansion and changes in EMC and also mediate organ specific metastasis during carcinogenesis [7;8]. Tumor metastatic potential can be determined by the tumor microenvironment and target organs [9;10].

Chemokine receptors are G protein coupled receptors and numerous cells show the expression of these receptors including leukocytes, endothelial cells, stromal cells, epithelial cells and tumor cells [10-12]. These receptors have vital roles in malignant tumor and cardiovascular diseases, also play role in allergic reactions, tissue damage and microbial infections [13;14]. Chemokine receptors are classified into four subfamilies on the basis of four subfamilies of chemokines they bind, CXCR, CCR, CX3CR and XCR.

Chemokine receptors play major role in tumor metastasis [14-16]. At each step of metastasis these receptors potentially facilitate tumor dissemination. In order to estimate the clinical significance of these receptors few clinical studies have been done. But there is no comprehensive study regarding all the chemokine receptors in NSCLC [17-19].

2. Expression of CXCL8 in NSCLC

In cancers having angiogenic phenotypes like NSCLC, CXCL8 is a very effective and powerful angiogenic factor. Its receptors are CXCR1 and CXCR2 [20].Tumor angiogenesis, metastasis and poor survival rate is related to high level of CXCL8 [21-23].

CXCL8 directly promotes proliferation of endothelial cell, chemo taxis and tubular morphogenesis [24-26]. CXCL8 was identified in a gene expression of patients that were predictive of poor prognosis with stage 1 lung cancer [7;27].

Two of the six cell lines of NSCLC expressed high levels of CXCL8, these cell lines are A549 and H441, while the other cell lines expressed low levels of CXCL8. Earlier studies assumed that only cancer cells produce CXCL8. However stromal cells secrete high level of CXCL8 and also increase tumor cells in tumor and stromal cells co-culture. Mechanism of this induction is still undefined. In several in-vitro models, cell to cell contact is involved in the induction of CXCL8 [20]. Role of CXCL8 in lung cancer is not obvious. CXCL8 receptors are present on lung cancerous cells but their effect on tumor angiogenesis and proliferation is still uncertain.

CXCR1 is a major receptor of CXCL8 which allows or influence the mitogenic activity of it in NSCLC. Thus, targeting mitogenic and angiogenic activity of CXCL8 may help to control tissue invasion and metastasis of NSCLC [20]. Circulating human CXCL8 can be a valuable, clinically applicable tumor protein marker owed to its affirmative correlation by means of numerous physiologic variables related by lung cancer progression.

3. Expression of CXCL5 & CXCL12 in NSCLC

CXCL5 is an important mediator of angiogenesis in NSCLC. In different experimental studies, it is observed that angiogenesis in NSCLC is directly correlated to higher level of CXCL5 [28].

Surgical specimens of NSCLC show a direct link between tumor angiogenesis and CXCL5. In SCID mice, CXCL5 expression was directly related to tumor proliferation and metastasis.

Reduction of CXCL5 expression, reduce tumor proliferation and metastases [28].This was also suggested by recent studies that the presence of CXCL5 in NSCLC have higher degree of correlation with both tumor proliferation and patient prognosis [21;29].

CXCL12 with CXCR4 had also been involved in stimulating angiogenesis of NSCLC [30;31]. However, recent experimental studies of NSCLC make it clear that CXCR4 is expressed on cancerous cells and does not stimulate tumor angiogenesis in an in vivo culture. In this experimental study, with reduction of CXCL12 level, no significant change in primary tumor size and tumor angiogenesis was observed [32].

However, there is an obvious reduction of metastasis of these tumors into *in vitro* culture, indicating that the CXCL12/CXCR4 promotes metastasis and proliferation of the tumor cells. A reason for this noticeable difference of these *in vivo* studies from other *in vitro* studies of angiogenesis mediated by CXCL12/CXCR4 is that CXCR4 expressing tumor cells can "outcompete" tumor-associated endothelial cells for CXCL12. Therefore, there is a very great difference in the function of CXCL12 against the other factors associated with angiogenesis, such that metastasis is promoted by CXCL5, CXCL8, and vascular endothelial growth factors.

CXCL5 & CXCL12 receptors over expression in tumor tissues possibly will suggest the development of diagnostic agents and therapy targeted at chemokine receptor-over expressing tumors. In this regard only some exhaustive clinical studies have been undertaken to assess the clinical importance of these receptors status but no comprehensive study has been known in NSCLC.

4. Expression of CXCR1& CXCR2

There are two cell surface receptors which bind to CXCL8, known as CXCR1 and CXCR2; these receptors have similar structure but different binding sites [33]. CXCR1 binds only with one CXC chemokine, CXCL8, while CXCR2 binds to numerous CXC chemokines. These receptors are present on different cell types including leukocytes, keratinocytes, endothelial cells [34;35] and various tumor cells including NSCLC[36;37].

When functions of CXCL8 and importance of its receptors, CXCR1 and CXCR2 were observed in different cancer cell lines, it was found that an increased level of CXCL8 mediated cell invasion and migration is directly correlated with increased expression of CXCR1 &CXCR2. By using different neutralizing antibodies, it was observed that CXCR1 was not involved in cell migration and invasion, only CXCR2 was involved, while both receptors are involved in angiogenesis. Thus making strategies against CXCL8 signaling pathways promises a better therapy of cancer. It is demonstrated by several studies that CXCR2 is responsible for CXCL8 mediated angiogenesis in NSCLC and human micro vascular endothelial cells [24;38;39].

CXCR1 is an important receptor which promotes the function of CXCL8. Thus targeting expression of CXCR1 & production of CXCL8 may ultimately help to develop strategies against lung cancer proliferation, invasion and metastasis.

5. Expression of CXCR4

CXCR4 is receptor for chemokine CXCL12. In NSCLC, tumor cells at stage 1 show expression of CXCR4, present in the nucleus and cytoplasm of these tumor cells. Several studies on tumor cells show that CXCR4 positive nuclear staining is related with improve survival rate. The 5 year overall survival rate was 93% for the patients having strong nuclear staining 52% for those having weak nuclear staining [10].

CXCL12 and its receptor CXCR4 promote metastasis of different tumors having angiogenic phenotype including NSCLC [17;32;40-42].CXCR4 may transform a benign tumor to malignant phenotype [17;43].

6. Expression of CXCR7

It was previously thought that CXCL12 has only one surface receptor, CXCR4, but Burns and colleagues [14;44] characterized that another receptor CXCR7 binds CXCL12. CXCR7 together with CXCR3 also has another ligand CXCL11. CXCR7 presents on many cell lines including cancer cell lines, fetal liver cells and activated endothelial cells. It facilitates angiogenesis and the blockage of CXCR7 inhibits tumor growth in mouse models.

Patients with EGFR gene mutations show high level of CXCR7 expression. Choi and colleagues reported that mutations in one EGFR domain, tyrosine kinase are responsible for phosphorylation of EGFR, tyrosine independent mutations and caused constant activation of EGFR [14;45].

Molecular analysis of tumor of patients that took part in the TRIBUT or IDEAL/INTAC experimental study revealed that patients with improve prognosis had an EGRF mutated tumor. This is one of the explanations that CXCR7 is an independent disease free prognostic factor [14].

Wang and colleagues by using qualitative mRNA characterized that increasing tumor grade show increased expression of CXCR7 in prostate cancer. Fluorescence activated cell sorting analysis also indicated higher CXCR7 expression [46].

In conclusion higher expression of CXCR7 is linked with tumor metastasis and poor survival of patients with P-stage1 NSCLC. As the elevated CXCR7 expression is directly correlated with increased EGFR gene mutations, therefore the expression of CXCR7 is not the only one factor for overall survival. We can also say that in future, studies of CXCR7 possibly will lead on the road to the development of diagnostic agents and targeted therapy for patients with p-stage I NSCLC.

7. Expression of receptors in tumor islets

Survival of NSCLC patients is directly related to CXCR2, CXCR3 and CXCR4 expression in tumor stroma. Expression of CXCR3 and CCR1 is also positively correlated to increase in number of mast cells and islet macrophages. The chemokine receptor CCR1 is present on macrophages and involved in the migration of macrophages into tumor islets. CCR1 is a receptor of CCL3 protein. TNF-α production and release is stimulated by CCL1 and has cytotoxic potential in tumor islets. Natural killer cells, T lymphocytes and mast cells show the expression of CXCR3; there is no evidence of expression of CXCR3 on macrophages [4;47-49]. These immune cells are linked with increase survival in NSCLC and together with macrophages involved tumor killing [4;19;50;51].

The tumors enriched for cells expressing CXCR3, having large quantities of one or all of the CXCR3 binding chemokines including CXCL9, CXCL10 and CXCL11. Host anti tumor immune response is mediated by expression of CXCR3 on various immune cells in mouse model. CXCR3 binding chemokines are secreted by a variety of inflammatory and structural cells and act as indicating markers for Th1 immunological [4;52].

In NSCLC, CCL5 produced by tumor epithelial cells and involved in determination of the nature and intensity of the immune response. While CXCR2 is not expressed in epithelial cells of the tumor islets, but is expressed on inflammatory cells. Expression of CXCR2 is directly correlated with increased survival. So it is suggested that neoplastic transformation is promoted by reduction of CXCR2 expression on epithelial cells in NSCLC. It is also suggested that expression of CXCR2 on inflammatory cells used to limit tumor proliferation. There is dichotomy in function of CXCR2 in NSCLC. In the stroma, it acts as an angiogenic factor and helps in tumor proliferation, but on the other side by the recruitment of the inflammatory cells to tumor islet, it limits tumor growth. Thus targeting CXCR2 has unpredictable effects depending on the relative balance between these two different functions [4].

Conclusively, this information can be considered to target the chemokines and chemokine receptors to establish the therapeutic strategies and to confine the tumor microenvironment to minimize the possibility of metastasis.

8. Acknowledgements

The authors are thankful to the Vice Chancellor of the University of the Punjab, Lahore, Pakistan for providing the financial assistance to meet the publication expenses.

9. References

[1] Bhattacharjee A, Richards WG, Staunton J et al. Classification of human lung carcinomas by mRNA expression profiling reveals distinct adenocarcinoma subclasses. Proc.Natl.Acad.Sci.U.S.A 2001;98:13790-13795.

[2] Jemal A, Siegel R, Ward E et al. Cancer statistics, 2007. CA Cancer J.Clin. 2007;57:43-66.

[3] Mulshine JL, Sullivan DC. Clinical practice. Lung cancer screening. N.Engl.J.Med. 2005;352:2714-2720.

[4] Ohri CM, Shikotra A, Green RH, Waller DA, Bradding P. Chemokine receptor expression in tumour islets and stroma in non-small cell lung cancer. BMC.Cancer 2010;10:172.

[5] Rossi D, Zlotnik A. The biology of chemokines and their receptors. Annu.Rev.Immunol. 2000;18:217-242.

[6] Slettenaar VI, Wilson JL. The chemokine network: a target in cancer biology? Adv.Drug Deliv.Rev. 2006;58:962-974.

[7] Baird AM, Gray SG, O'Byrne KJ. Epigenetics underpinning the regulation of the CXC (ELR+) chemokines in non-small cell lung cancer. PLoS.One. 2011;6:e14593.

[8] Lazennec G, Richmond A. Chemokines and chemokine receptors: new insights into cancer-related inflammation. Trends Mol.Med. 2010;16:133-144.

[9] Balkwill F. Cancer and the chemokine network. Nat.Rev.Cancer 2004;4:540-550.

[10] Reckamp KL, Figlin RA, Burdick MD et al. CXCR4 expression on circulating pan-cytokeratin positive cells is associated with survival in patients with advanced non-small cell lung cancer. BMC.Cancer 2009;9:213.

[11] Kakinuma T, Hwang ST. Chemokines, chemokine receptors, and cancer metastasis. J.Leukoc.Biol. 2006;79:639-651.
[12] Zlotnik A, Yoshie O. Chemokines: a new classification system and their role in immunity. Immunity. 2000;12:121-127.
[13] Coussens LM, Werb Z. Inflammation and cancer. Nature 2002;420:860-867.
[14] Iwakiri S, Mino N, Takahashi T et al. Higher expression of chemokine receptor CXCR7 is linked to early and metastatic recurrence in pathological stage I nonsmall cell lung cancer. Cancer 2009;115:2580-2593.
[15] Rollins BJ. Chemokines. Blood 1997;90:909-928.
[16] Taub DD. Chemokine-leukocyte interactions. The voodoo that they do so well. Cytokine Growth Factor Rev. 1996;7:355-376.
[17] Spano JP, Andre F, Morat L et al. Chemokine receptor CXCR4 and early-stage non-small cell lung cancer: pattern of expression and correlation with outcome. Ann.Oncol. 2004;15:613-617.
[18] Su L, Zhang J, Xu H et al. Differential expression of CXCR4 is associated with the metastatic potential of human non-small cell lung cancer cells. Clin.Cancer Res. 2005;11:8273-8280.
[19] Takanami I. Overexpression of CCR7 mRNA in nonsmall cell lung cancer: correlation with lymph node metastasis. Int.J.Cancer 2003;105:186-189.
[20] Zhu YM, Webster SJ, Flower D, Woll PJ. Interleukin-8/CXCL8 is a growth factor for human lung cancer cells. Br.J.Cancer 2004;91:1970-1976.
[21] Chen JJ, Yao PL, Yuan A et al. Up-regulation of tumor interleukin-8 expression by infiltrating macrophages: its correlation with tumor angiogenesis and patient survival in non-small cell lung cancer. Clin.Cancer Res. 2003;9:729-737.
[22] Masuya D, Huang C, Liu D et al. The intratumoral expression of vascular endothelial growth factor and interleukin-8 associated with angiogenesis in nonsmall cell lung carcinoma patients. Cancer 2001;92:2628-2638.
[23] Yuan A, Yang PC, Yu CJ et al. Interleukin-8 messenger ribonucleic acid expression correlates with tumor progression, tumor angiogenesis, patient survival, and timing of relapse in non-small-cell lung cancer. Am.J.Respir.Crit Care Med. 2000;162:1957-1963.
[24] Anderson IC, Mari SE, Broderick RJ, Mari BP, Shipp MA. The angiogenic factor interleukin 8 is induced in non-small cell lung cancer/pulmonary fibroblast cocultures. Cancer Res. 2000;60:269-272.
[25] Koch AE, Polverini PJ, Kunkel SL et al. Interleukin-8 as a macrophage-derived mediator of angiogenesis. Science 1992;258:1798-1801.
[26] Kumar R, Yoneda J, Bucana CD, Fidler IJ. Regulation of distinct steps of angiogenesis by different angiogenic molecules. Int.J.Oncol. 1998;12:749-757.
[27] Seike M, Yanaihara N, Bowman ED et al. Use of a cytokine gene expression signature in lung adenocarcinoma and the surrounding tissue as a prognostic classifier. J.Natl.Cancer Inst. 2007;99:1257-1269.
[28] Arenberg DA, Keane MP, DiGiovine B et al. Epithelial-neutrophil activating peptide (ENA-78) is an important angiogenic factor in non-small cell lung cancer. J.Clin.Invest 1998;102:465-472.

[29] White ES, Flaherty KR, Carskadon S et al. Macrophage migration inhibitory factor and CXC chemokine expression in non-small cell lung cancer: role in angiogenesis and prognosis. Clin.Cancer Res. 2003;9:853-860.
[30] Bachelder RE, Wendt MA, Mercurio AM. Vascular endothelial growth factor promotes breast carcinoma invasion in an autocrine manner by regulating the chemokine receptor CXCR4. Cancer Res. 2002;62:7203-7206.
[31] Salcedo R, Wasserman K, Young HA et al. Vascular endothelial growth factor and basic fibroblast growth factor induce expression of CXCR4 on human endothelial cells: In vivo neovascularization induced by stromal-derived factor-1alpha. Am.J.Pathol. 1999;154:1125-1135.
[32] Phillips RJ, Burdick MD, Lutz M et al. The stromal derived factor-1/CXCL12-CXC chemokine receptor 4 biological axis in non-small cell lung cancer metastases. Am.J.Respir.Crit Care Med. 2003;167:1676-1686.
[33] Cerretti DP, Kozlosky CJ, Vanden Bos T et al. Molecular characterization of receptors for human interleukin-8, GRO/melanoma growth-stimulatory activity and neutrophil activating peptide-2. Mol.Immunol. 1993;30:359-367.
[34] Cataisson C, Ohman R, Patel G et al. Inducible cutaneous inflammation reveals a protumorigenic role for keratinocyte CXCR2 in skin carcinogenesis. Cancer Res. 2009;69:319-328.
[35] Richardson RM, Marjoram RJ, Barak LS, Snyderman R. Role of the cytoplasmic tails of CXCR1 and CXCR2 in mediating leukocyte migration, activation, and regulation. J.Immunol. 2003;170:2904-2911.
[36] Norgauer J, Metzner B, Schraufstatter I. Expression and growth-promoting function of the IL-8 receptor beta in human melanoma cells. J.Immunol. 1996;156:1132-1137.
[37] Varney ML, Li A, Dave BJ et al. Expression of CXCR1 and CXCR2 receptors in malignant melanoma with different metastatic potential and their role in interleukin-8 (CXCL-8)-mediated modulation of metastatic phenotype. Clin.Exp.Metastasis 2003;20:723-731.
[38] Heidemann J, Ogawa H, Dwinell MB et al. Angiogenic effects of interleukin 8 (CXCL8) in human intestinal microvascular endothelial cells are mediated by CXCR2. J.Biol.Chem. 2003;278:8508-8515.
[39] Salcedo R, Resau JH, Halverson D et al. Differential expression and responsiveness of chemokine receptors (CXCR1-3) by human microvascular endothelial cells and umbilical vein endothelial cells. FASEB J. 2000;14:2055-2064.
[40] Burger JA, Kipps TJ. CXCR4: a key receptor in the crosstalk between tumor cells and their microenvironment. Blood 2006;107:1761-1767.
[41] Muller A, Homey B, Soto H et al. Involvement of chemokine receptors in breast cancer metastasis. Nature 2001;410:50-56.
[42] Phillips RJ, Mestas J, Gharaee-Kermani M et al. Epidermal Growth Factor and Hypoxia-induced Expression of CXC Chemokine Receptor 4 on Non-small Cell Lung Cancer Cells Is Regulated by the Phosphatidylinositol 3-Kinase/PTEN/AKT/Mammalian Target of Rapamycin Signaling Pathway and Activation of Hypoxia Inducible Factor-1+¦. Journal of Biological Chemistry 2005;280:22473-22481.
[43] Holland JD, Kochetkova M, Akekawatchai C et al. Differential functional activation of chemokine receptor CXCR4 is mediated by G proteins in breast cancer cells. Cancer Res. 2006;66:4117-4124.

[44] Burns JM, Summers BC, Wang Y et al. A novel chemokine receptor for SDF-1 and I-TAC involved in cell survival, cell adhesion, and tumor development. J.Exp.Med. 2006;203:2201-2213.

[45] Choi SH, Mendrola JM, Lemmon MA. EGF-independent activation of cell-surface EGF receptors harboring mutations found in gefitinib-sensitive lung cancer. Oncogene 2007;26:1567-1576.

[46] Wang J, Shiozawa Y, Wang J et al. The role of CXCR7/RDC1 as a chemokine receptor for CXCL12/SDF-1 in prostate cancer. J.Biol.Chem. 2008;283:4283-4294.

[47] Brightling CE, Kaur D, Berger P et al. Differential expression of CCR3 and CXCR3 by human lung and bone marrow-derived mast cells: implications for tissue mast cell migration. J.Leukoc.Biol. 2005;77:759-766.

[48] Newton P, O'Boyle G, Jenkins Y, Ali S, Kirby JA. T cell extravasation: demonstration of synergy between activation of CXCR3 and the T cell receptor. Mol.Immunol. 2009;47:485-492.

[49] Wendel M, Galani IE, Suri-Payer E, Cerwenka A. Natural killer cell accumulation in tumors is dependent on IFN-gamma and CXCR3 ligands. Cancer Res. 2008;68:8437-8445.

[50] Villegas FR, Coca S, Villarrubia VG et al. Prognostic significance of tumor infiltrating natural killer cells subset CD57 in patients with squamous cell lung cancer. Lung Cancer 2002;35:23-28.

[51] Welsh TJ, Green RH, Richardson D et al. Macrophage and mast-cell invasion of tumor cell islets confers a marked survival advantage in non-small-cell lung cancer. J.Clin.Oncol. 2005;23:8959-8967.

[52] Matsuda A, Fukuda S, Matsumoto K, Saito H. Th1/Th2 cytokines reciprocally regulate in vitro pulmonary angiogenesis via CXC chemokine synthesis. Am.J.Respir.Cell Mol.Biol. 2008;38:168-175.

7

Treatment of Breast Cancer: New Approaches

Nadeem Sheikh*, Saba Shehzadi and Arfa Batool
Department of Zoology, University of the Punjab, Q-A campus, Lahore Pakistan

1. Introduction

Breast cancer is the most common type of malignancy in the world and is also one of the major reasons of mortality among women worldwide. It exhibits a vast variety of pathological features and clinical signs and said to be a heterogeneous disease (Jemal *et al.*, 2009). It is also among the most studied cancers, but the biology of it is still not well understood (Fang *et al.*, 2011). Genetics, inheritance, aging are major risk factors for breast cancer, while hormonal factors, obesity (imitating in diet and exercise), and alcohol use presenting more diffident risk. Breast cancer mortality has been found to be decreasing gradually since 1990s, after the improvement of breast cancer screening techniques and the advancement of treatment approaches (Jatoi and Miller, 2003; and Tabar *et al.*, 2003).

1.1 Incidence of breast cancer in Pakistan

In Pakistan, breast cancer has maximum prevalence of all types of cancer, with frequencies similar to Western population. It affects mostly young women (45 or above) in Pakistan with a high frequency as compared to Caucasian women (Kakarala *et al.*, 2010), often presenting in advanced stage (Malik, 2002). The low socio-economic status and reproductive issues such as low parity and late first pregnancy may be responsible for higher incidence of breast cancer in Pakistan. It is described that patients with lower socio-economic status (SES) had larger, more aggressive tumors with worsened survival outcomes (Aziz *et al.*, 2010). The mutations of *BRCA1* and *BRCA2* genes are also considered as responsible factors for the greater numbers of breast cancer in Pakistan. As Pakistan has the maximum number of consanguineous marriages in the world (Hashmi, 1997), the transfer of these mutations after such marriages is supposed to be a vital factor in raising breast cancer cases in Pakistan (Shami *et al.*, 1991). The inheritance of recessive genes has been reported to increase the breast cancer risk in Pakistan (Liede *et al.*, 2002). But the exact reasons for high incidence of breast cancer in Pakistan are still to be detected.

All these risks put an emphasis on the development of better treatment strategies for breast cancer. Early finding of diseased condition, improvements in scientific methodologies and quality of care, with sufficient economic guidelines, need to be developed for countries with limited resources like Pakistan (Aziz *et al.*, 2008).

---

* Corresponding Author

2. Biological explanation of breast cancer

Breast cancer usually arises after menopause (age: 40+), but it can also arise before menopause in very rare cases. The ovarian-pituitary axis synchronizes the normal breast physiology during the reproductive cycle. The biological reason for it is that the glandular component of the breast gradually degenerates after menopause and the breast is mostly substituted by adipose tissue. Any problem in this process causes the development of breast cancer, whereas by epithelial cells of the breast ducts, uncontrolled growth and survival takes place, and in later stages the characteristics of neo-angiogenesis, invasion and metastasis occurs (Heldermon and Ellis, 2006).

3. Treatment and prevention

Breast cancer prevention is primarily made by pharmacoprevention using fenretinide and tamoxifen. The regular use of screening techniques for early detection of breast cancer is the best strategy to decrease death rates (Veronesi and Boyle, 1993). Better treatments include targeted chemotherapy, endocrine therapy, radiotherapy and surgery, inhibitors of certain proteins and more recently immune therapy (monoclonal antibodies) and miRNA therapy. Advancement in life style may also be a good treatment for breast cancer. Breast cancer threat may be reduced by physical activities or exercise (Eliassen *et al.*, 2010).

Many targeted genetic and molecular agents have been developed for efficient treatment of breast cancer, by keeping in view certain biomolecular characteristics of breast cancer, such as mutations of breast cancer susceptibility gene type 1, 2 (BRCA1/BRCA2) (Chen and Parmigiani, 2007), abnormal activation of human epidermal growth factor receptors (EFGR) (Wang and greene, 2007), overexpression of human epidermal growth factor receptor-2 (HER-2) (Ross *et al.*, 2003), and activation of vascular endothelial growth factor (VEGF) receptor (Bhinder and Ramaswamy, 2010). It is reported that more than half of the breast cancer cases are due to errors in hormone receptor proteins. For this reason, the primary concern of today's research is endocrine therapy. The development of targeting molecular agents is also among major goals of current research for efficient treatment of advanced breast cancer.

The major obstacles in treatment of breast cancer are resistance to therapeutic agents (Serrano-Olvera *et al.*, 2006). Women with breast cancer treatment and surgery have complaints of tension and depression. By using different treatment strategies including mastectomy, adjuvant chemotherapy, many women have shown incidence of nervousness and depression associated with cancer that puts unpleasant effects on the life status and emotional working.

3.1 Chemotherapy

Chemotherapy is the most primitive method for treating breast cancer, if employed immediately after surgery, termed as adjuvant chemotherapy (AC), and administered before surgery, neoadjuvant chemotherapy (NAC) (Alvarado-Cabrero *et al.*, 2009). Chemotherapy is recommended for all women with invasive cancer greater than 1 centimeter (Ganz *et al.*, 2011). Adjuvant chemotherapy is associated with significantly more severe physical symptoms, including musculo-skeletal pain, vaginal and weight problems and nausea (Ganz *et al.*, 2011).

3.1.1 Neoadjuvant chemotherapy

Neoadjuvant chemotherapy (NAC) has been a common approach for the management and treatment of locally advanced breast cancer (LABC). It is applied very effectively for treatment of patients with LABC before breast and axillary lymph node resection (Pusztai, 2008). The NAC is aimed to reduce tumor size subsequently aiding mastectomy and radiotherapy (Cleator *et al.*, 2002; and Pusztai, 2008). NAC is better treatment option because it averts adverse physiological reactions (Alvarado-Cabrero *et al.*, 2009).

Patients of LABC had showed complete clinical and pathological response to NAC, while those with pure micropapillary carcinoma (PMC) gave incomplete response (Alvarado-Cabrero *et al.*, 2009). Patient's therapy effect can be predicted by clinical & pathological responses (Jones *et al.*, 2006), and by biomarker levels in the patients, which have better prognostic influence in contrast to pathological and clinical response, multi-biomarker levels have showed better expressive power for treatment outcome as compared with single biomarker level (Nolen *et al.*, 2008).

Paclitaxel is a chemical agent applied before radiotherapy and surgery. It binds to tubulin resulting in cell cycle arrest at M-phase which enhances radiation sensitivity. In a report, Patients having 3 cycles of paclitaxel followed by simultaneous radiotherapy before specific surgery, showed better results as compared those without paclitaxel (Chakravarthy *et al.*, 2000). The most common approach for treating LABC in developed countries consists of NAC with anthracyclines and taxanes followed by surgery and radiation therapy (Osako *et al.*, 2007). HR-positive tumors are less chemosensitive so an anthracyline based NAC is developed without hormonal treatment to evaluate estrogen receptor (ER) and progesterone receptor (PgR) semi-quantitative expression in patients with HR-positive tumors (Petit *et al.*, 2010). Preoperative and postoperative marker studies in NAC might facilitate tumor analysis and to observe possible change in status respectively (Piper *et al.*, 2004).

3.2 Endocrine therapy

An understanding of the mechanism of action, pharmacology and clinical indications for various classes of endocrine agent is critical for the management of breast cancer (Heldermon and Ellis, 2006). Breast cancer is divided into three major molecular types which are diagnosed by routine histopathological tests: (i) hormone receptor-positive (ER/PR+), (ii) human epidermal growth factor receptor type 2 enriched (HER2+) and (iii) triple negative (ER-, PR-, HER2-) breast cancer (TNBC). HR+ breast cancers comprise about 60–70% of all the clinically positive breast cancers, while the other two types equally accounts for the remaining 30–40% of all breast cancer cases (Slamon *et al.*, 1989). Endocrine therapy has been used before surgery but Dittmer *et al.*, (2011) reported adjuvant endocrine therapy not so effective for breast tumor treatment because of its side effects (Dittmer *et al.*, 2011).

3.2.1 HER2+ breast cancer and targeted therapy

The HER2 overexpression due to gene amplification or transcriptional deregulation (Slamon *et* al., 1989) presents a poorer prognosis, with development of resistance to many chemotherapeutic and hormonal agents, and a rise in tendency of metastasis to brain (Serrano-Olvera *et al.*, 2006).

3.2.2 Monoclonal antibodies for endocrine therapy

The basic purpose of current therapeutic policies is to make overexpressed HER2 silent with certain targeted complexes e.g., trastuzumab, a monoclonal antibody prepared for humans against HER2 protein, reported to be a well accepted therapy for women with MBC (Vogel *et al.,* 2002). This antibody specifically hinders the HER2-mediated activation of intracellular kinases and other molecules (Valabrega *et al.,* 2007). The combination of chemotherapy and trastuzumab extends the life of patient in adjuvant and metastatic patterns, but most women with HER2+ metastatic tumor become resistant to trastuzumab; about 15–25% of women detected with early HER2+ disease have trastuzumab-resistant tumors (Bedard *et al.,* 2009).

The combinations of anti-HER2 agents should close to abolish acquired drug resistance, shorten the period of therapy, and potentially dole out with the need of coexisting chemotherapy, because the anti-HER2 therapies including drugs trastuzumab and lapatinib, targeted against the HER2 signaling network has gradually changed the natural history of early and metastatic HER2-overexpressing breast cancer (Abramason and Artega, 2011).

3.2.3 HR+ breast cancer and targeted therapy

Estrogen is a well-characterized growth factor in about 60–70% of breast cancer patients (Clemons and Goss, 2001). The malignant epithelial cells depend on reproductive hormones, specifically estrogen in ER+ tumors (Heldermon and Ellis, 2006). The initial endocrine therapy of breast cancer was removal of the ovaries (oophorectomy) (Taylor *et al.,* 1998). Many thriving remedies have been formulated to decrease or eradicate circulating estrogen or to obstruct its communication with genomic target objects. The specific ER antagonist tamoxifen is recommended as adjuvant endocrine therapy for the hormone receptor positive early breast cancer (Sehdev *et al.,* 2009). Endocrine therapies for ER+ patients include three types of agents that (i) directly target ER through molecules that bind ER and change ER function; (ii) estrogen deprivation through aromatase inhibition or ovarian suppression; and (iii) sex steroid therapies, including estrogen, progestins and androgens.

3.2.4 Selective Estrogen Receptor Modulators (SERM)

The rise of estrogen level in blood proposed the use of a therapeutic modulator to oestrogen, a selective oestrogen receptor modulator, or SERM (Jordan, 1999). The evidences from breast cancer treatment trials presented the ability of the first SERM, tamoxifen, to avoid tumors in the contralateral breast of women receiving adjuvant therapy (Ragaz and Coldman, 1998). Tamoxifen considerably lessens the rate of treatment failure in breast cancer patients, with lesser frequency of clinically obvious toxic effects. For tamoxifen, response rates range from 16 to 56%, and an improved toxicity profile than alternative therapies, for example large dosage of estrogen or adrenalectomy results in quick acceptance of tamoxifen as a selective cure for advanced disease (Muss *et al.,* 1994). The combination of ovarian suppression and tamoxifen is referred to as the first line therapy for HR+ advanced breast cancer in pre-menopausal women. Some examples of SERM comprise raloxifene and toremifine (Holli *et al.,* 2000; and Martino *et al.,* 2004).

3.2.5 Tyrosine kinase inhibitors

Lapatinib is an oral, selective, reversible small-molecule dual tyrosine kinase inhibitor of both the ErbB1 and ErbB2 signaling pathway that works by inhibiting growth and guiding to cell arrest and apoptosis. It is presented to be effective against HER-2+, LABC and metastatic breast cancer (MBC). The primary activity of lapatinib in breast cancer patients is mediated through HER-2 inhibition. In addition, lapatinib treatment inhibits the growth of ErbB2-overexpressing human breast cancer cells that showed resistance to trastuzumab. Clinically related antitumor activity has not been reported when lapatinib is used in the mixed population of LABC patients with distinct HER-2 negative or HER-2 untested tumors (Leo *et al.,* 2008). Patients with HER-2 negative or HER-2 untested MBC had not showed any advantage from lapatinib therapy. However, the first-line therapy with paclitaxel and lapatinib in combination expressed improved clinical outcomes in HER-2+ patients. Future assessment of the effectiveness and safety of this combination is constant in early and metastatic HER-2+ breast cancer patients. A combined targeted approach with letrozole and lapatinib has appreciably improved progression free survival in patients with MBC that coexpresses HR and HER2.

3.2.6 Triple-negative breast cancer treatment

CCN1, also known as Cyr61 (cysteine-rich 61), is a proangiogenic factor, increased CCN1 expression is associated with the development of tumors (O'Kelly *et al.,* 2008), e.g., in about 30% of invasive breast carcinomas, and particularly in triple-negative breast carcinomas (TNBC). TNBCs patients had been treated with bisphosphonate in combination to chemotherapy. Zoledronic acid (ZOL) is a bisphosphonate having direct antitumor activity in breast tumor cells by preventing independent growth, branching and morphogenesis by targeting CCN1 overexpressing cells through a negative regulation of CCN1 by FOXO3a; it is a new therapeutic approach for TNBC (Espinoza *et al.,* 2011).

3.3 Anti-angiogenic therapies

Angiogenesis is the mandatory step in tumor development, so anti-angiogenic agents can be developed for the better management and prevention of breast tumor. The monoclonal antibody to platelet/endothelial cell adhesion molecule (PECAM) has proved to be a sensitive and specific marker for endothelial cells; these antibodies might reduce the tumor size or hinder the development of metastatic tumors (Horak *et al.,* 1992).

3.3.1 Viral vector therapy

Expression of VEGF in several types of tumors is amplified, subsequently correlated with weak prognosis of several tumors. Im *et al* (2001) used transfection method to create a replication-deficient adenoviral vector containing antisense VEGF cDNA (Ad5CMV-αVEGF) to down-regulate VEGF expression. This therapeutic strategy notably repressed the growth of developed breast tumors (Im *et al.,* 2001). These viral vectors may be used in future for targeting the tumor vasculature in breast cancer therapy.

3.4 Surgery

Mastectomy is total removal of one or both breasts; it is frequently used in treatment of invasive breast cancers in early stages (Veronesi *et al.,* 2002). Bilateral mastectomy is effective therapeutic approach for breast cancers with BRCA1 and BRCA2 mutations (Meijers-Heijboer *et al.,* 2001). Lumpectomy or breast conserving surgery (i.e., surgical removal of discrete tumor from breast) may be used alone or in combination with subsequent radiotherapy, later is reported to be more appropriate therapy for invasive breast cancer; because the risk of ipsilateral recurrence of breast cancer is very low in lumpectomy with irradiation as compared with mastectomy and lumpectomy alone (Fisher *et al.,* 2002). For hormone receptor positive breast cancer, initial treatment option was surgical removal of ovaries, oophorectomy (Taylor *et al.,* 1998).

3.5 Radiotherapy

Radiotherapy is applied after surgery, i.e., adjuvant radiotherapy. Cardiovascular disease continues to be chief problem of radiotherapy in breast cancer patients, but a little is known about it yet; It raises the enduring threat for cardiovascular mortality, predominantly in women treated for left-sided breast cancer; the mortality rate due to cardiac disease may boost to double in left-sided breast cancer survivors as compared to right-sided breast cancer patients (Foody, 2011). In women (aged 70+) with tumors larger than 5 cm, minor local regional recurrence (LRR) was observed through radiotherapy following mastectomy than those lacking radiotherapy (Truong *et al.,* 2005); Post-mastectomy radiotherapy (PMRT) might be helpful in the managing breast cancer with high-risk features (Lee *et al.,* 2005). Adjuvant radiotherapy is proved to be a breast conserving therapy (BCT) in younger women, it is not frequently recommended for patients with older age (Nagel *et al.,* 2002). Postoperative radiotherapy is normally in use for treating patients with positive surgical margins following mastectomy but a little data is present to sustain this approach (Truong *et al.,* 2004).

3.6 miRNA therapy

Each tumor type seems to have a unique miRNA marker, and such markers are being oppressed to recognize the tissue of origin of metastatic tumors and to distinguish between different cancer subtypes (Lu *et al.,* 2005). Furthermore, miRNA expression markers are linked to numerous clinicopathological features for instance tumor stage, receptor status and patient survival. Eventually, it is likely to make profiles that characterize a probable link between circulating miRNAs, disease status, basic subtype and HER2+ status, therapeutic response and metastatic risk. As miRNA expression is vanished during MBC, the renovation of these miRNAs' expression may suppress MBC; for example, miR-126 renovation reported to decrease in general tumor growth and propagation, and miR-335 presented to inhibit metastatic cell invasion (Tavazoie *et al.,* 2008).

3.7 Male breast cancer and treatment

Breast cancer is recently described to exist in males too. Tamoxifen, aromatase inhibitors and GnRH analogues targeting on HER2-directed therapies, PARP inhibitors, and angiogenesis inhibitors are reported endocrine therapeutic strategies for treating male breast cancer (Onami *et al.,* 2010).

4. Conclusion

Breast cancer is a heterogeneous disease and has become the most common cancer in women throughout the world. Known risk factors include age, dietary features, reproductive hormonal imbalance, genetic predispositions, alcoholism, and breast adipose tissue density. Breast cancer is major cause of mortality of women worldwide. Keeping in view the above discussion, here is a need of developing better therapeutic plans for hampering breast cancer risks and reducing mortality due to breast cancer. Research investigating cultural, environmental, and genetic issues of breast cancer should be taken into consideration for development of better treatment plans and to present additional details for the clinical and pathological features. The molecular, endocrine and genetic means should be the major goals of today's efforts for treatment of breast cancer.

5. Acknowledgements

The authors are thankful to the Vice Chancellor of the University of the Punjab, Lahore, Pakistan for providing the financial assistance to meet the publication expenses.

6. References

Abramason, V. and Artega, C.L., 2011. New Strategies in HER2-Overexpressing Breast Cancer: Many Combinations of Targeted Drugs Available. *Clin Cancer Res.,* 17:952–8.

Alvarado-Cabrero, I., Alderete-Vázquez, G., Quintal-Ramírez, M., Patiño, M. and Ruíz, E., 2009. Incidence of pathologic complete response in women treated with preoperative chemotherapy for locally advanced breast cancer: correlation of histology, hormone receptor status, Her2/Neu, and gross pathologic findings. *Annals of Diagnostic Pathology,* 13:151–7.

Aziz, Z., Iqbal, J. and Akram, M., 2008. Predictive and prognostic factors associated with survival outcomes in patients with stage I-III breast cancer: A report from a developing country. *Asian Pacific J Clin Oncol.,* 4:81-90.

Aziz, Z., Iqbal, J., Akram, M. and Anderson, B.O., 2010. Worsened oncologic outcomes for women of lower socio-economic status (SES) treated for locally advanced breast cancer (LABC) in Pakistan. *The Breast,* 19:38-43.

Bedard, P.L., De Azambuja, E. and Cardoso, F., 2009. Beyond trastuzumab: overcoming resistance to targeted HER-2 therapy in breast cancer. *Curr Cancer Drug Targets,* 9:148–62.

Bhinder, A., Carothers, S. and Ramaswamy, B., 2010.Antiangiogenesis Therapy in Breast Cancer. *Current Breast Cancer Reports,* 2:4-15.

Chakravarthy, A., Nicholsan, B., Kelley, M., Beauchamp, D., Johnson, D., Frexes-Steed, M., Simpson, J., Shyr, Y. and Pietenpol, J., 2000. A pilot study of neoadjuvant paclitaxel and radiation with correlative molecular studies in stage II/III breast cancer. *Clin Breast Cancer,* 1:68-71.

Chen, S. and Parmigiani, G., 2007. Meta-analysis of BRCA1 and BRCA2 penetrance. *J Clin Oncol.,* 25:1329-33.

Cleator, S., Parton, M. and Dowsett, M., 2002. The biology of neoadjuvant chemotherapy for breast cancer. *Endocr Relat Cancer,* 9:183–95.

Clemons, M. and Goss, P., 2001. Estrogen and the risk of breast cancer. *N Engl J Med.,* 344(4):276-85.

Dittmer, C., Roeder, K., Hoellen, F., Salehin, D., Thill, M. and Fischer, D., 2011. Compliance to adjuvant therapy in breast cancer patients. *Eur J Gynaecol Oncol.,* 32:280-2.

Eliassen, A.H., Hankinson, S.E., Rosner, B., Holmes, M.D. and Willett, W.C., 2010. Physical activity and risk of breast cancer among postmenopausal women. *Arch. Intern. Med.*, 170(19):1758–64.

Espinoza, I., Liu, H., Buspy, R. and Lupu, R., 2011. CCN1, a Candidate Target for Zoledronic Acid Treatment in Breast Cancer. *Mol Cancer Ther.*, 10:732-41.

Fang, F., Turcan,S., Rimner,A., Kaufman,A., Giri,D., Morris,L.G.T., Shen,R., Seshan,V., Mo,Q., Heguy,A., Baylin,S.B., Ahuja,N., Viale,A., Massague,J., Norton,L., Vahdat,L.T., Moynahan,M.E. and Chan,T.A., 2011.Breast Cancer Methylomes Establish an Epigenomic Foundation for Metastasis. *Sci Transl Med.*, 3:75.

Fisher, B., Anderson, S., Bryant, J., Margolese, R.G., Deutsch, M., Fisher, E.R., Jeong, J.H. and Wolmark, N., 2002. Twenty-year follow-up of a randomized trial comparing total mastectomy, lumpectomy, and lumpectomy plus irradiation for the treatment of invasive breast cancer. *N Engl J Med.*, 347(16):1233-41.

Foody, J.M., 2011. Radiotherapy for Breast Cancer and Cardiovascular Mortality. *Journal Watch Cardiology.*

Ganz, P.A., Kwan, L., Stanton, A.L., Bower, J.E. and Belin, R.T., 2011. Physical and Psychosocial Recovery in the Year after Primary Treatment of Breast Cancer. *Am Soc Clin Oncol.*, 29:1101-9.

Hashmi, M., 1997. Frequency of consanguinity and its effect on congenital malformation--a hospital based study. *J Pak Med Assoc.*, 47:75–8.

Heldermon, C. and Ellis, M., 2006. Endocrine Therapy for Breast Cancer. *Update on Cancer Therapeutics*, 1:285-97.

Holli, K., Valavaara, R., Blanco, G., *et al.*, Safety and efficacy results of a randomized trial comparing adjuvant toremifene and tamoxifen in postmenopausal patients with node-positive breast cancer. Finnish Breast Cancer Group. *J Clin Oncol.*, 18(20):3487–94.

Horak, E.R., Klenk, N., Leek, R., Lejeune, S., Smith, K., Stuart, N., Harris, A.L., Greenall, M. and Stepniewska, K., 1992. Angiogenesis assessed by platelet/endothelial cell adhesion molecule antibodies, as indicator of node metastases and survival in breast cancer. *Lancet*, 340:1120-4.

Im, S.A., Kim, J.S., Manzano, C.G., Fueyo, J., Liu, T.J., Cho, M.S., Seong, C.M., Lee, S.N., Hong, Y.K. and Yung,W.K.A., 2001. Inhibition of breast cancer growth in vivo by antiangiogenesis gene therapy with adenovirus-mediated antisense-VEGF. *Br J Cancer*, 84:1252–7.

Jatoi, I. and Miller, A.B., 2003. Why is breast-cancer mortality declining? *Lancet Oncol.*, 4:251–4.

Jemal, A., Siegel, R., Ward, E., Hao, Y., Xu, J. and Thun, M.J., 2009. Cancer Statistics. *CA Cancer J Clin.*, 59:225-49.

Jordan, V.C., 1999. Breast cancer prevention in the primary care setting. *Primary Care & Cancer*, 19:9–10.

Jones, R.L., Lakhani, S.R., Ring, A.E., *et al.*, 2006. Pathological complete response and residual DCIS following neoadjuvant chemotherapy for breast carcinoma. *Br J Cancer*, 94:358-62.

Kakarala, M., Rozek, L., Cote, M., Liyanage, S. and Brenner, D.E., 2010 Breast cancer histology and receptor status characterization in Asian Indian and Pakistani women in the U.S. - a SEER analysis. *BMC Cancer*, 10:191.

Lee, J.C., Truong, P.T., Kader, H.A., Speers, C.H. and Olivotto, I.A., 2005. Postmastectomy radiotherapy reduces locoregional recurrence in elderly women with high-risk breast cancer. *Clin Oncol (R Coll Radiol).*, 17:623-9.

Leo, A.D., Gomez, H.L., Aziz, Z., Zvirbule, Z., Bines, J., Arbushites, M.C., Guerrera, S.F., Koehler,M., Oliva, C., Stein, S.H., Williams, L.S., Dering, J., Finn,R.S. and Press, M.F., 2008. Phase III, Double-Blind, Randomized Study Comparing Lapatinib Plus Paclitaxel With Placebo Plus Paclitaxel As First-Line Treatment for Metastatic Breast Cancer. *J Clin Oncol.*, 26(34): 5544-5552.

Liede, A., Malik, I.A., Aziz, Z., De Los Rios, P., Kwan, E. and Narod, S.A., 2002. Contribution of BRCA1 and BRCA2 Mutations to Breast and Ovarian Cancer in Pakistan. *Am J Hum Genet.*, 71: 595-606.

Lu, J., Getz, G., Miska, E.A., Alvarez-Saavedra, E., Lamb, J., Peck, D., Sweet-Cordero, A., Ebert Bl., Mak Rh., Ferrando, A.A., Downing, J.R., Jacks, T., Horvitz, H.R. and Golub, T.R., 2005. MicroRNA expression profiles classify human cancers. *Nature,* 9:834-8.

Malik, I.A., 2002. Clinico-pathological features of breast cancer in Pakistan. *J Pak Med Assoc.,* 52:100–4.

Martino, S., Cauley, J.A., Barrett-Connor, E., *et al.,* 2004. Continuing outcomes relevant to Evista: breast cancer incidence in postmenopausal osteoporotic women in a randomized trial of raloxifene. *J Natl Cancer Inst.,* 96(23):1751–61.

Meijers-Heijboer, H., Van Geel, B., Van Putten, W.L. *et al.,* 2001. Breast cancer after prophylactic bilateral mastectomy in women with BRCA1 and BRCA2 mutations. *N Engl J Med.,* 345(3):159–164.

Muss, H.B., Case, L.D., Atkins, J.N., *et al.,* 1994. Tamoxifen versus high-dose oral medroxyprogesterone acetate as initial endocrine therapy for patients with metastatic breast cancer: a piedmont oncology association study. *J Clin Oncol.,* 12(8):1630–8.

Nagel, G., Röhrig, B., Hoyer, H., Füller, J. and Katenkamp, D., 2002. A population-based study on variations in the use of adjuvant radiotherapy in breast cancer patients. *Strahlenther Onkol..* 178:589-96.

Nolen, B.M., Marks, J.R., Tasan, S., Rand, A., Luong, T.M., Wang, Y., Blackwell, K. and Lokshin, A.E., 2008. Serum biomarker profiles and response to neoadjuvant chemotherapy for locally advanced breast cancer. *Breast Cancer Res.,* 10(3):45.

O'kelly, J., Chung, A., Lemp, N., Chumakova, K., Yin, D.G., Wang H., Said J., Gui, D., Miller, C.W., Karlan, B.Y. and Koeffler, H.P., 2008. Functional domains of CCN1 (Cyr61) regulate breast cancer progression. *Int J Oncol.,* 33(1):59-67.

Onami, S., Ozaki, M., Mortimer, J.E. and Pal, S.K., 2010. Erratum to Male breast cancer: An update in diagnosis, treatment and molecular profiling. *Maturitas,* 65:308-14.

Osako, T., Horii, R., Matsuura, M., Ogiya, A., Domoto, K., Miyagi, Y., Takahashi, S., Ito, Y., Iwase, T. and Akiyama, F., 2007. Common and discriminative clinicopathological features between breast cancers with pathological complete response or progressive disease in response to neoadjuvant chemotherapy. *J Cancer Res Clin Oncol.,* 136:233-41.

Petit, T., Wilt, M., Velten, M., Rodier, J.F., Fricker, J.P., Dufour, P. and Ghnassia, J.P., 2010. Semi-quantitative evaluation of estrogen receptor expression is a strong predictive factor of pathological complete response after anthracycline-based neo-adjuvant chemotherapy in hormonal-sensitive breast cancer. *Breast Cancer Res Treat.,* 124:387-91.

Piper, G.L., Patel, N.A., Patel, J.A., Malay, M.B. and Julian, T.B., 2004. Neoadjuvant chemotherapy for locally advanced breast cancer results in alterations in preoperative tumor marker status. *Am Surg.,* 70:1103-6.

Pusztai, L., 2008. Preoperative systemic chemotherapy and pathologic assessment of response. *Pathol Oncol Res.,* 14:169-71.

Ragaz, J. and Coldman, A., 1998. Survival impact of adjuvant tamoxifen on competing causes of mortality in breast cancer survivors, with analysis of mortality from contralateral breast cancer, cardiovascular events, endometrial cancer, and thromboembolic episodes. *J Clin Oncol.,* 16:2018–24.

Ross, J.S., Fletcher, J.A., Linette, G.P., Stec, J., Clark, E., Ayers, M., Symmans, W.F., Pusztai, L. and Bloom, K.J., 2003. The Her-2/neu gene and protein in breast cancer 2003: biomarker and target of therapy. *Oncologist,* 8:307–25.

Sehdev, S., Martin, G., Sideris, L., Lam, W. and Brisson, S., 2009. Safety of adjuvant endocrine therapies in hormone receptor-positive early breast cancer. *Curr Oncol.,* 16:14-23.

Serrano-Olvera, A., Dueñas-González, A., Gallardo-Rincón, D., Candelaria, M. and Garza-Salazar, J.D., 2006. Prognostic, predictive and therapeutic implications of HER2 in invasive epithelial ovarian cancer. *Cancer Treat Rev.,* 32:180–90.

Shami, S.A., Qaisar, R. and Bittles, A.H., 1991.Consanguinity and adult morbidity in Pakistan. *Lancet,* 338:954–5.

Slamon, D.J., Godolphin, W., Jones, L.A., Holt, J.A., Wong, S.G., Keith, D.E., Levin, W.J., Stuart, S.G., Udove, J., Ullrich, A. *et al.,* 1989. Studies of the HER-2/neu proto-oncogene in human breast and ovarian cancer. *Science,* 244:707–12.

Tabar, L., Yen, M.F. and Vitak, B., 2003. Mammography service screening and mortality in breast cancer patients: 20-year follow-up before and after introduction of screening. *Lancet*, 361:1405–10.

Tavazoie, S.F., Alarcón, C., Oskarsson, T., Padua, D., Wang, Q., Bos, P.D., Gerald, W.L. and Massagué, J., 2008. Endogenous human microRNAs that suppress breast cancer metastasis. *Nature*, 451:147-52.

Taylor, C.W., Green, S., Dalton, W.S., Martino, S., Rector, D., Ingle, J.N., Robert, N.J., Budd, G.T., Paradelo, J.C., Natale, R.B., Bearden, J.D., Mailliardj, A. and Osborne, C.K., 1998. Multicenter randomized clinical trial of goserelin versus surgical ovariectomy in premenopausal patients with receptor-positive metastatic breast cancer: an intergroup study. *J Clin Oncol.*, 16:994-9.

Truong, P.T., Olivotto, I.A., Speers, C.H., Wai, E.S., Berthelet, E. and Kader, H.A., 2004. A positive margin is not always an indication for radiotherapy after mastectomy in early breast cancer. *Int J Radiat Oncol Biol Phys.*, 58(3):797-804.

Truong, P.T., Lee, J., Kader, H.A., Speers, C.H. and Olivotto, I.A., 2005. Locoregional recurrence risks in elderly breast cancer patients treated with mastectomy without adjuvant radiotherapy. *Eur J Cancer.*, 41:1267-77.

Vogel, C.L., Cobleigh, M.A., Tripathy, D., Gutheil, J.C., Harris, L.N., Fehrenbacher, L., Slamon, D.J., Murphy, M., Novotny, W.F., Burchmore, M., Shak, S., Stewart, S.J. and Press, M., 2002. Efficacy and safety of trastuzumab as a single agent in first-line treatment of HER2-overexpressing metastatic breast cancer. *J Clin Oncol.,* 20(3):719-26.

Valabrega, G., Montemurro, F. and Aglietta, M., 2007. Trastuzumab: mechanism of action, resistance and future perspectives in HER2-overexpressing breast cancer. *Ann Oncol.,* 18:977–84.

Veronesi, U. and Boyle, P., 1993. Breast Cancer. *Eur J Cancer,* 29(10):1410-4.

Veronesi, U., Cascinelli, N., Mariani, L., *et al.,* 2002. Twenty Year Follow Up of a randomized study comparing breast conserving surgery with radical (Halsted) mastectomy for early breast cancer. *N Engl J Med.,* 347:1227-32.

Wang, Q. and Greene, M.I., 2007. The development of targeted therapy in the ErbB system. *Am Soc Clin Oncol.,Ed Book:*79-84.